The Bilingual Mind

COGNITION AND LANGUAGE

A Series in Psycholinguistics • Series Editor: R. W. RIEBER

Recent Volumes in this Series:

THE BILINGUAL MIND:
Thinking, Feeling and Speaking in Two Languages
Rafael Art. Javier

THE COLLECTED WORKS OF L. S. VYGOTSKY
Volume 1: Problems of General Psychology
Volume 2: The Fundamentals of Defectology (Abnormal Psychology and Learning Disabilities)
Volume 3: Problems of the Theory and History of Psychology
Volume 4: The History of the Development of Higher Mental Functions
Volume 5: Child Psychology
Volume 6: Scientific Legacy

EXPERIMENTAL SLIPS AND HUMAN ERROR:
Exploring and Architecture of Volition
Edited by Bernard J. Baars

LANGUAGE FOR THOSE WHO HAVE NOTHING
Mikhail Bakhtin and the Landscape of Psychiatry
Peter Good

LANGUAGE, THOUGHT, AND THE BRAIN
Tatyana B. Glezerman and Victoria I. Balkoski

PSYCHOENVIRONMENTAL FORCES IN SUBSTANCE ABUSE PREVENTION
Lorand B. Szalay, Jean Bryson Strohl, and Kathleen T. Doherty

THE PSYCHOPATHOLOGY OF LANGUAGE AND COGNITION
Robert W. Rieber and Harold J. Vetter

TIME, WILL, AND MENTAL PROCESS
Jason W. Brown

VYGOTSKY'S PSYCHOLOGY-PHILOSOPHY: A Metaphor for Language Theory and Learning
Dorothy Robbins

VYGOTSKY'S SOCIOHISTORICAL PSYCHOLOGY AND ITS CONTEMPORARY APPLICATIONS
Carl Ratner

Rafael Art. Javier

The Bilingual Mind

Thinking, Feeling and Speaking in Two Languages

Springer

Rafael Art. Javier
St. John's University
8000 Utopian Parkway
Queens, New York 11439
USA
Tel: (718) 990-5460 or 1972
Fax: (718) 990-5485
javierr@stjohns.edu

Library of Congress Control Number: 2007921193

ISBN 978-0-387-30913-2 e-ISBN 978-0-387-30914-9

Printed on acid-free paper.

9 8 7 6 5 4 3 2 1

springer.com

To my son, Joshua
An invitation to continue solidifying his bilingual and bicultural identity

Island

bewitched
space time
Mother
flying manatees
coconuts that play
black rhythms
hanging ripe mangoes
waiting to be sucked
through that infinitesimal
seeping life-giving
hole
parrot fish
gently dancing dazzle
with their brilliant colors
I baptize myself deep
in your inviting warm
turquoise blue waters
I discover my origins
prior to sex and conscience
innocent clear
I feel I float
in your amniotic fluid
you feed me and I exist
yesterday today tomorrow
I breathe you I drink you
in a frigid
January morning
de mi lindo *Nueva York*
your tropical air
warms my
being
and once again
I am
thinking feeling
speaking
en *español*

Alina Camacho-Gingerich, Ph.D.

Acknowledgment

This book is the result of several years of gestation where the determination of producing a different kind of book than normally written was the guiding force. To the extent to which this was accomplished, my thanks go to Robert Rieber, a friend and mentor who over the years encouraged me, in subtle and more direct ways, to complete the book. But my passion for bilingualism was sparked at the Millhauser Lab, New York University Medical Center, where I had the fortune to meet and work closely with Dr. Murray Alpert and Dr. Luis Marcos who were already engaged in bilingual research and welcomed me to their labs with open arms. For their guidance over the years, I thank them. Some of my students were instrumental in some aspects of this book, like Dr. Michele Munoz, who worked in some of the research projects discussed in the book, and Lorie Blas, who worked hard and extended herself to make possible the completion of the book within the time frame. I thank them both. I also extend my thanks to Clare Douglas who assisted me in the midst of her hectic day to find language distribution maps and scan material needed for the book. My former secretary, Cathy Lancellotti, should also be thanked for helping me to keep the office going while I was the Director of the Center for Psychological Services and Clinical Studies at St. John's University and making it possible for me to focus on working on the book. Margaret Cashin's assistance is also greatly appreciated for helping me find important material that I needed for the book. Her unwavering willingness to search for difficult-to-find documents and her excellent computer skills made it easier for me to complete this book project within reasonable time. Thank you. I also want to thank my patients for illuminating me on how bilingualism affected their lives and how it gave them their unique texture, quality, and flavor that was different than the other patients. The poem "Island" by Dr. Camacho-Gingerich included in this book was specifically selected not only for its literary merit but because it clearly illustrates the subject matter of the book. I thank Dr. Camacho-Gingerich for her important contribution. She read and provided important suggestions in some sections of the book. Finally, I would like to thank my son, Joshua, to whom I am dedicating this book. It is a great and humbling experience to see him slowly growing as a Latino young man with his dual heritage (Latino/Irish-American).

Contents

1
Bilingualism and Social Context: An Introduction

It is clear by now that bilingualism is an inescapable fact of life both in the United States and abroad. The interaction of different linguistic groups has been made more commonplace by the fluidity of the political and economic conditions in many countries, as well as the rapid changes in computer technology and worldwide telecommunication network. But unlike previous factors that encouraged language contacts through a physical interaction among individuals from different linguistic communities, as described by Mackey (1967) and Grosjean (1982), this time, no physical immigration is necessary for language contacts to take place. Indeed, the world has been made quite small with the proliferation of the Internet and other means of communication that have made possible the easy interaction among the many linguistic communities of the world. For instance, one can easily watch or listen to news and programs transmitted in French, British English, Greek, Italian, Chinese, Spanish, etc., with actual images from the respective countries that provide the listener/viewer with unique perspectives of the world events that cannot be obtained any other way. Similarly, foreign films have increasingly become part of the art world made more possible, in part, by the proliferation of internet and cable television programs even in, so called, underdeveloped countries. These films are generally produced in specific countries in which native languages are spoken by native speakers, thus providing the listener/viewer with cultural, linguistic, and ecological contacts from specific countries, without the individual physically immigrating to these countries.

Nevertheless, immigration in the traditional manner continues to occur as individuals continue to feel compelled to take the extraordinary steps to uproot themselves from their familiar cultural and linguistic groups and immigrate to different cultural and linguistic communities. The reasons for these have remained the same over the course of the years because, in the final analysis, it has to do with the individual's fundamental search for a better, more meaningful, safer, and more productive life condition. Thus, one may decide to immigrate for social or economic reasons, for trade and commerce, for political and religious reasons, and/or for educational and cultural reasons (Baca & Javier, 1995; Grosjean, 1982; Javier, 2002; Mackey, 1967); the end result is the cultural and linguistic clashes that characterize the lives of many immigrants, and that, under the best of circumstances, finally lead to bilingualism.

For bilingualism to occur, the individual has to find clear social, political, economic, educational, and/or professional advantages. The host country also has to maintain a policy of encouragement and tolerance, which has not always been the case throughout the world. Examples of antagonistic attitudes against minority languages in the United States are amply discussed by Grosjean in his 1982 book "Life with Two Languages." These include the results of the 1980 election in which the voters of Dade County, Florida, repealed a 1973 statute that made the county officially bilingual in English and Spanish. Also in the 1980s, a federal court in Texas upheld an earlier decision that allowed an employer to forbid the use of minority languages among employees in the workplace. The same pattern is also seen in the educational system where the bilingual education has been under severe attack.

It is quite different in Europe and other countries where it is not unusual to encounter individuals having a command of two or three languages. That does not mean, however, that the relationship between and among the linguistic communities in these countries is totally harmonious. Part of the reason for this is the fact that language is often connected to national pride and political and economic positions. As Prial described in his 1980 *New York Times* article on April 22 regarding the language and political problem in Belgium, "it was not just economy that brought down the Martens government. It was also language, a problem that has troubled this small nation since its creation in 1830" (p. 2). About one half of the people speak Dutch (called Flemings) and the rest speak French (called Walloons) and yet another group also speak a form of low German, especially at home. The tension has been so great that a proposal was made to turn Belgium into a kind of federal state with three autonomous regions: Flanders, Wallonia, and Brussels (French-speaking). This notwithstanding, the majority of the population can speak both of the dominant languages, with the understanding that French is still the key to success.

In the United States, the view that bilingualism causes more problems in the educational system than it is worth has culminated in proposals such as Proposition 227 in California in 1998 and Proposition 203 in Arizona, in November 2000, calling for the elimination of all bilingual programs and a substantial reduction of federal, state, and city funding for bilingual education. For instance, during President Reagan's administration, services offered to minorities, such as bilingual education, experienced substantial cuts in federal funding (Grosjean, 1982). In New York City, bilingual education has also been under severe scrutiny, especially during Giuliani's administration, with a strong recommendation to revamp all the existent bilingual programs.

Linguistic Communities

This notwithstanding, the possibility for interacting with different linguistic and cultural communities is quite overwhelming when we consider the enormous number of different languages spoken in the world. According to Grosjean

(1982), there are around 4,000 languages in the world in about 150 countries. According to statistics published by SIL International, the number is much greater, with 6,912 known living languages (www.ethnologue.com, retrieved 7/16/06). The fact of the matter is that interacting with individuals from different linguistic and cultural backgrounds is a common occurrence in many metropolitan cities around the world and, becoming progressively so, in many sectors in the United States. To drive this point home, let's look at the census data, including the most recent census.

In the United States alone, non-English-speaking communities are present in many regions, as shown in the language maps published by www.ethnologue.com and www.mla.org/census_map depicting the linguistic distributions in all the regions of the United States. In fact, the 1976 survey statistics already show strong non-English-speaking communities in six basic regions:

New Mexico	44%
Hawaii	35%
California	25%
Texas	25%
New York City	25%
Arizona	23%

But the linguistic diversity in the United States is very extensive, including languages that are not regularly referred to in normal discourse. See, for instance, the different linguistic communities depicted in Tables 1.1–1.7 and Figures 1.1–1.6.

These table and figures give the reader a good idea of the enormous diversity of languages in many regions of the United States, languages most prominent in the United States, and the areas where we are most likely to find the largest concentration of these languages. They also give the reader a good sense of the percentage of speakers of a specific language as compared with the total population of speakers and bilingual speakers in the specific region being examined. Although we only included more specific language information pertaining to New York, New Jersey, Pennsylvania, Texas, New Mexico and Wisconsin, when we analyze the language distributions in the whole United States, the following facts emerge (Grosjean, 1982; Lehrer & Sloan, 2005; www.ethnologue.com; www.mla.org/census_map):

- Spanish is found in many areas, with the largest concentration in Arizona, California, Colorado, New Mexico, Texas, and New York.
- German is found in Pennsylvania, California, Illinois, and north central regions.
- French is found in Louisiana, Massachusetts, and New York.
- Italian is found in New York, New Jersey, Pennsylvania, northern states, Illinois, and California.

- Polish is found in northeastern and north central states (New Jersey/ Illinois/Michigan).
- Scandinavian is found in Minnesota, Iowa, and the Dakotas.
- Chinese is found in California, New York, and Massachusetts.
- Japanese is found in California.
- Korean is found in California and Maryland.
- Vietnamese is found in California and Maryland.
- Creole is found in New York, Florida and Massachusetts.

TABLE 1.1. Breakdown of the subcategories of various languages spoken in the United States based on the 2000 US census.

Linguistic groups	Subclassification	Examples
Spanish:	Spanish	Spanish
	Spanish Creole	Ladino
Other Indo-European languages:	French	French, Cajun, Patois
	French Creole	Haitian Creole
	Italian	
	Portuguese	Portuguese
	Portuguese Creole	Papia Mentae
	German	
	Yiddish	
	Other West Germanic languages:	Dutch, Pennsylvania Dutch, Afrikaans
	Scandinavian Languages	Danish, Norwegian, Swedish
	Greek	
	Russian	
	Polish	
	Serbo-Croatian	Serbo-Croatian, Croatian, Serbian
	Other Slavic languages:	Czech, Slovak Ukrainian
	Armenian	
	Persian	
	Gujarati	
	Hindi	
	Urdu	
	Other Indic languages:	Bengali, Marathi, Punjabi, Romany
	Other Indo-European languages:	Albanian, Gaelic, Lithuanian, Rumanian
Asian and Pacific Island languages	Chinese	Cantonese, Formosan, Mandarin
	Japanese	
	Korean	
	Mon-Khmer, Cambodian	
	Miao, Hmong	
	Thai	
	Loatian	
	Vietnamese	
	Other Asian languages:	Dravidian languages (Malayalam, Telugu, Tamil), Turkish

	Tagalog	
	Other Pacific Island languages:	Chamorro, Hawaiian, Ilocano, Indonesian, Samoan
Other languages	Navajo	
	Other Native North American languages:	Apache, Cherokee, Dakota, Pima, Yupik
	Hungarian	
	Arabic	
	Hebrew	
	African languages	Amharic, Ibo, Twi, Yoruba, Bantu, Swahili, Somali
	Other languages:	Syriac, Finnish

TABLE 1.2. Age breakdown of languages spoken in New York with percentage of each language spoken as compared with all languages spoken in New York.

Languages	Ages 5–17	18–64	65 +	Total	Percent
English	2,518,325	8,380,590	1,887,275	12,786,190	72.04
All languages other than English combined	927,946	3,470,416	563,018	4,961,380	27.96
Spanish	540,245	1,713,850	161,945	2,416,040	13.61
Chinese	47,710	223,865	32,585	304,160	1.71
Italian	20,650	170,085	103,530	294,265	1.65
Russian	31,750	147,945	39,070	218,765	1.23
French	27,150	124,435	22,495	174,080	0.98
French Creole	24,580	80,800	9,365	114,745	0.64
Yiddish	36,460	51,520	25,535	113,515	0.63
Polish	11,675	67,410	32,645	111,730	0.62
Korean	16,485	78,455	7,170	102,110	0.57
German	7,525	55,895	29,260	92,680	0.52
Greek	10,185	60,165	16,310	86,660	0.48
Arabic	14,155	50,990	4,810	69,955	0.39
Hebrew	14,735	47,385	5,555	67,675	0.38
Tagalog	6,490	52,870	6,140	65,500	0.36
Urdu	13,170	37,610	1,665	52,445	0.29
Bengali	10,850	39,555	1,360	51,765	0.29
Cantonese	6,580	30,865	4,605	42,050	0.23
Portuguese	5,815	32,025	3,480	41,320	0.23
Hindi	5,605	33,445	2,105	41,155	0.23
Japanese	3,655	29,090	1,820	34,565	0.19
Kru, Ibo, Yoruba	5,310	28,040	700	34,050	0.19
Albanian	6,660	18,695	1,275	26,630	0.15
Persian	5,205	18,410	2,355	25,970	0.14
Ukrainian	3,140	13,350	6,875	23,365	0.13
Punjabi	4,935	16,830	795	22,560	0.12
Vietnamese	3,750	15,545	955	20,250	0.11
Malayalam	3,500	14,950	820	19,270	0.10
Mandarin	2,620	15,185	1,235	19,040	0.10
Hungarian	970	9,785	7,665	18,420	0.10
Totals	**3,446,271**	**11,851,006**	**2,450,293**	**17,747,570**	

TABLE 1.3. Age breakdown of languages spoken in New Jersey with percentage of each language spoken as compared with all languages spoken in New Jersey.

Languages	Ages 5–17	18–64	65 +	Total	Percent
English	1,156,705	3,791,380	906,490	5,854,575	74.53
All languages other than English combined	366,185	1,427,882	206,165	2,000,232	25.49
Spanish	211,245	700,970	55,480	967,695	12.31
Italian	7,850	66,055	42,460	116,365	1.48
Polish	9,145	46,205	19,310	74,660	0.95
Portuguese	12,780	55,975	4,070	72,825	0.92
Tagalog	7,820	53,345	5,690	66,855	0.85
Chinese	11,685	49,735	5,000	66,420	0.84
Korean	11,510	40,990	2,835	55,335	0.70
Gujarati	9,070	35,260	2,995	47,325	0.60
Arabic	10,640	33,280	3,135	47,055	0.59
French	7,530	33,350	4,795	45,675	0.58
German	2,935	23,830	14,235	41,000	0.52
Russian	6,140	26,945	5,480	38,565	0.49
Hindi	3,895	26,425	1,080	31,400	0.39
French Creole	7,115	20,395	1,270	28,780	0.36
Greek	3,075	18,535	4,955	26,565	0.33
Urdu	4,725	13,370	640	18,735	0.23
Hebrew	3,640	10,195	1,160	14,995	0.19
Kru, Ibo, Yoruba	2,455	12,190	320	14,965	0.19
Vietnamese	2,305	10,435	570	13,310	0.16
Japanese	2,050	9,360	1,030	12,440	0.15
Hungarian	665	6,015	4,545	11,225	0.14
Ukrainian	990	6,565	3,670	11,225	0.14
Indian (not elsewhere classified)	1,575	7,975	480	10,030	0.12
Bengali	2,180	7,470	340	9,990	0.12
Turkish	1,845	7,425	490	9,760	0.12
Yiddish	1,075	3,015	5,055	9,145	0.11
Telugu	975	7,970	185	9,130	0.11
Tamil	990	6,675	260	7,925	0.10
Punjabi	1,605	5,640	485	7,730	0.09
Totals	**1,522,890**	**5,219,262**	**1,112,655**	**7,854,807**	

TABLE 1.4. Age breakdown of languages spoken in Pennsylvania with percentage of each language spoken as compared with all languages spoken in Pennsylvania.

Languages	Ages 5–17	18–64	65 +	Total	Percent
English	2,003,585	6,803,475	1,775,995	10,583,055	91.59
All languages other than English combined	189,346	637,799	144,044	971,189	8.41
Spanish	92,890	247,075	16,775	356,740	3.08
Italian	4,845	35,515	30,075	70,435	0.60
German	11,460	41,455	15,750	68,665	0.59
French	9,695	32,170	5,035	46,900	0.40
Pennsylvania Dutch	10,680	20,685	8,245	39,610	0.34
Chinese	5,815	27,435	2,295	35,545	0.30
Russian	5,490	20,800	5,900	32,190	0.27

Polish	2,400	12,985	16,330	31,715	0.27
Korean	4,730	19,660	1,590	25,980	0.22
Vietnamese	5,320	19,405	1,155	25,880	0.22
Arabic	3,965	13,880	1,715	19,560	0.16
Greek	1,845	11,365	4,135	17,345	0.15
Ukrainian	1,265	5,975	4,865	12,105	0.10
Dutch	2,565	6,470	1,825	10,860	0.09
Hindi	1,270	8,565	210	10,045	0.08
Tagalog	760	8,010	840	9,610	0.08
Gujarati	1,510	6,985	460	8,955	0.07
Slovak	320	2,240	6,260	8,820	0.07
Mon-Khmer, Cambodian	2,945	5,430	335	8,710	0.07
Portuguese	1,290	6,375	645	8,310	0.07
Japanese	845	5,550	810	7,205	0.06
Hungarian	380	2,955	2,825	6,160	0.05
Hebrew	1,330	4,085	504	5,919	0.05
Malayalam	1,135	4,500	220	5,855	0.05
Yiddish	145	1,420	3,880	5,445	0.04
Urdu	1,345	3,510	210	5,065	0.04
French Creole	1,320	3,335	130	4,785	0.04
Indian (not elsewhere classified)	810	3,515	185	4,510	0.03
Serbo-Croatian	930	2,480	825	4,235	0.03
Totals	**2,192,931**	**7,441,274**	**1,920,039**	**11,554,244**	

TABLE 1.5. Age breakdown of languages spoken in Texas with percentage of each language spoken as compared with all languages spoken in Texas.

Languages	Ages 5–17	18–64	65 +	Total	Percent
English	2,882,740	8,692,390	1,655,635	13,230,765	68.77
All languages other than English combined	1,380,393	4,217,201	411,498	6,009,092	31.23
Spanish	1,254,270	3,604,095	336,815	5,195,180	27.00
Vietnamese	25,025	91,400	6,095	122,520	0.63
German	8,680	56,320	17,100	82,100	0.42
Chinese	12,465	55,230	4,895	72,590	0.37
French	7,985	43,810	8,755	60,550	0.31
Tagalog	4,500	32,470	3,010	39,980	0.20
Korean	6,465	30,130	1,860	38,455	0.19
Urdu	7,490	24,315	1,175	32,980	0.17
Arabic	6,420	24,765	1,725	32,910	0.17
Hindi	2,485	17,735	700	20,920	0.10
Kru, Ibo, Yoruba	2,720	16,635	365	19,720	0.10
Gujarati	3,095	15,035	1,010	19,140	0.09
Persian	3,005	13,585	965	17,555	0.09
Japanese	1,780	10,880	2,040	14,700	0.07
Malayalam	2,500	10,070	465	13,035	0.06
Czech	460	5,050	7,295	12,805	0.06
Russian	1,735	8,550	1,290	11,575	0.06
Italian	630	8,080	2,445	11,155	0.05
Laotian	2,355	7,675	340	10,370	0.05
Portuguese	1,690	7,470	505	9,665	0.05

(*Continued*)

TABLE 1.5. (*Continued*)

Languages	Ages 5–17	18–64	65 +	Total	Percent
Polish	1,015	5,885	2,755	9,655	0.05
Mon-Khmer, Cambodian	1,900	5,715	260	7,875	0.04
Telugu	780	6,600	190	7,570	0.03
Bengali	1,255	6,120	175	7,550	0.03
Mandarin	1,285	5,840	215	7,340	0.03
Thai	690	6,465	130	7,285	0.03
Amharic	865	5,675	65	6,605	0.03
Greek	685	4,755	1,130	6,570	0.03
Tamil	580	5,315	105	6,000	0.03
Totals	**4,263,133**	**12,909,591**	**2,067,133**	**19,239,857**	

TABLE 1.6. Age breakdown of languages spoken in New Mexico with percentage of each language spoken as compared with all languages spoken in New Mexico.

Languages	Ages 5–17	18–64	65 +	Total	Percent
English	260,215	673,070	139,660	1,072,945	63.54
All languages other than English combined	117,803	425,270	72,561	615,634	36.46
Spanish	91,945	334,205	59,535	485,685	28.76
Navajo	15,400	47,940	5,450	68,790	4.07
Keres	2,420	6,790	1,085	10,295	0.60
German	855	5,695	1,325	7,875	0.46
Zuni	1,855	4,355	370	6,580	0.38
French	540	3,080	675	4,295	0.25
Tewa	630	2,090	495	3,215	0.19
Chinese	490	1,895	145	2,530	0.14
Vietnamese	405	1,955	165	2,525	0.14
Tiwa	340	1,375	240	1,955	0.11
Italian	150	1,125	660	1,935	0.11
Towa	560	1,220	129	1,909	0.11
Tagalog	160	1,305	140	1,605	0.09
Japanese	105	810	345	1,260	0.07
Korean	215	900	80	1,195	0.07
Arabic	165	735	80	980	0.05
Apache	164	700	70	934	0.05
Persian	90	585	70	745	0.04
Russian	99	575	50	724	0.04
Greek	100	400	220	720	0.04
Polish	85	384	205	674	0.03
Dutch	49	430	190	669	0.03
Jicarilla	49	515	84	648	0.03
Portuguese	134	455	50	639	0.03
Gujarati	105	360		465	0.02
Thai	29	390		419	0.02
Hebrew	75	265	35	375	0.02
Hindi	30	344		374	0.02
Laotian	110	250		360	0.02
Totals	**378,018**	**1,098,340**	**212,221**	**1,688,579**	

TABLE 1.7. Age breakdown of languages spoken in Wisconsin with percentage of each language spoken as compared with all languages spoken in Wisconsin.

Languages	Ages 5–17	18–64	65 +	Total	Percent
English	938,880	3,056,810	657,675	4,653,365	92.68
All languages other than English combined	86,470	236,433	44,741	367,644	7.32
Spanish	44,720	117,645	6,415	168,780	3.36
German	7,960	26,420	13,925	48,305	0.96
Miao, Hmong	15,445	14,145	980	30,570	0.60
French	4,000	9,450	1,410	14,860	0.29
Polish	815	5,200	6,080	12,095	0.24
Italian	415	4,040	2,320	6,775	0.13
Chinese	945	5,210	405	6,560	0.13
Russian	700	3,840	825	5,365	0.10
Arabic	830	3,030	225	4,085	0.08
Korean	745	3,155	170	4,070	0.08
Norwegian	255	1,255	2,010	3,520	0.07
Laotian	1,035	2,150	125	3,310	0.06
Vietnamese	705	2,410	100	3,215	0.06
Japanese	480	2,250	455	3,185	0.06
Tagalog	230	2,635	275	3,140	0.06
Dutch	600	1,725	780	3,105	0.06
Serbian	355	1,905	555	2,815	0.05
Greek	179	1,660	730	2,569	0.05
Pennsylvania Dutch	1,010	1,440	99	2,549	0.05
Hindi	200	1,945	145	2,290	0.04
Czech	110	690	935	1,735	0.03
Urdu	465	1,225	24	1,714	0.03
Albanian	335	970	65	1,370	0.02
Swedish	85	590	610	1,285	0.02
Finnish	129	505	650	1,284	0.02
Ojibwa	305	845	90	1,240	0.02
Winnebago	290	800	124	1,214	0.02
Punjabi	120	1,045		1,165	0.02
Serbo-Croatian	225	645	275	1,145	0.02
Totals	**1,025,350**	**3,293,243**	**702,416**	**5,021,009**	

The 2000 census further confirms the proliferation of languages found on the US soil, revealing even more pronouncedly the unique cultural and linguistic fabric of the American culture as a land of immigrants and linguistic diversity. See, for instance, a 3/8/02 *New York Times* article "A Little Russia on the Hudson" (p. E1) describing Russian enclaves or Russian influences now proliferating more and more around New York City. Thus, we can now find Russian-speaking immigrants in Brighton Beach, Brooklyn, Rego Park (Queens), Midtown Manhattan, and Soho. It is their way to develop a version of Russian life in America, and in the process they manage to influence the American cuisine and art in tangible ways. For instance, the Russian Tea Room was an institution

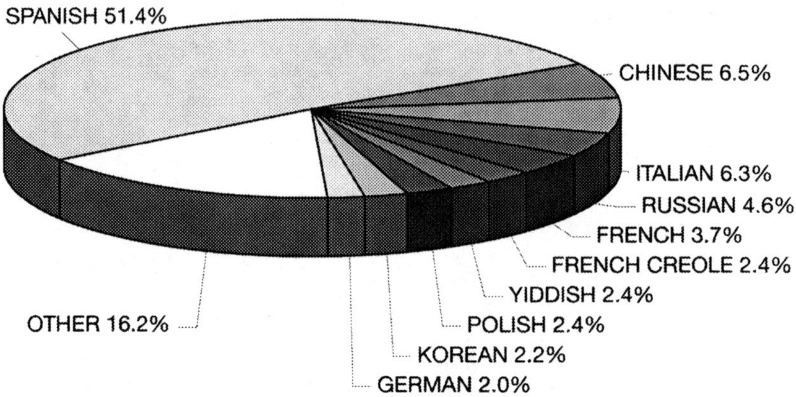

FIGURE 1.1. Pie depiction of the most spoken languages in New York.

until its closing; the Firebird and Russian Samovar in Manhattan and La Brioche Café in Brighton Beach, continue to be favorite eating places for many.

But let's take another look at Table 1.1 to get a better picture of the enormous linguistic diversity in the United States (US Census 2000). The data in Table 1.1 refer only to the languages spoken at home. Persons who knew other languages but did not use them at home were excluded from this calculation. Thus, the total percentage of bilinguals in the United States may be even greater than that offered by these statistics. Four basic linguistic group classifications were identified: Spanish, other Indo-European languages, Asian and Pacific Island languages, and other languages, each with several languages represented.

One can see that about 321 different languages are found in the United States alone, distributed among the different linguistic classifications. The concern has been that the more linguistically diverse the immigrant population in the United States becomes, the more the danger that English will loose its primacy as the language of choice. But this concern is not supported by the most recent statistics

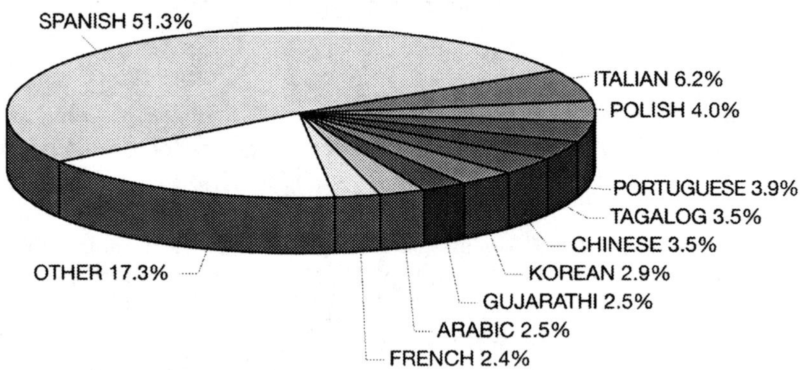

FIGURE 1.2. Pie depiction of the most spoken languages in New Jersey.

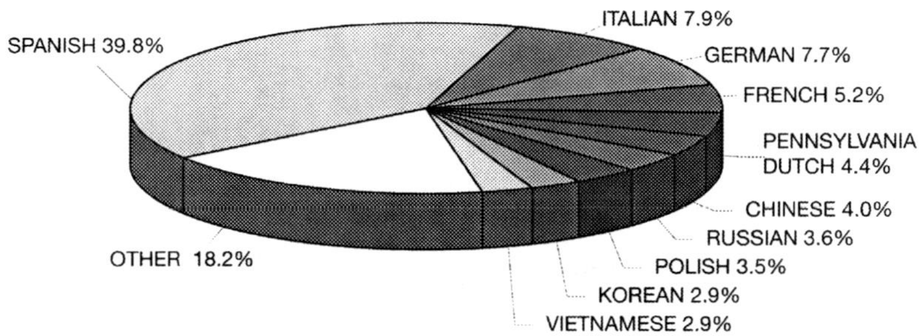

FIGURE 1.3. Pie depiction of the most spoken languages in Pennsylvania.

(US Census, 2000), considering the increasing percentage of immigrants who reported different degrees of linguistic proficiency in English. For instance, of the 254,746,174 estimated total US population, 44,304,495 speak other languages. Of those who speak other languages, a significant number maintains a language proficiency in English as well (Table 1.8). This is particularly the case with younger immigrants, but it is also a pattern found in the older population. In the case of younger immigrants, of the total 9,733,738 linguistically diverse immigrants between the ages of 5 and 17 years, 69% reported speaking English "very well" and 19% reported speaking English "well." Similar patterns can be seen in immigrants between the ages of 18 and 64. Of the total 31,094,270 immigrants in this age range, 54% reported speaking English "very well" and 21% reported speaking it "well."

The United States is, indeed, a nation of immigrants, a fact that was recently reaffirmed in response to the World Trade Center disaster. The census data presented reflect the rapid changes in the face of North America (US Census 2000), with its members now coming in larger numbers from Latin America and the Caribbean countries, Asia, the Middle East, and the old Soviet Union. This

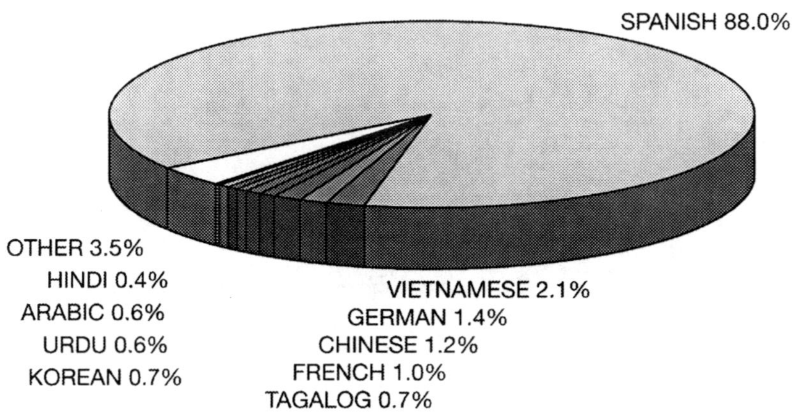

FIGURE 1.4. Pie depiction of the most spoken languages in Texas.

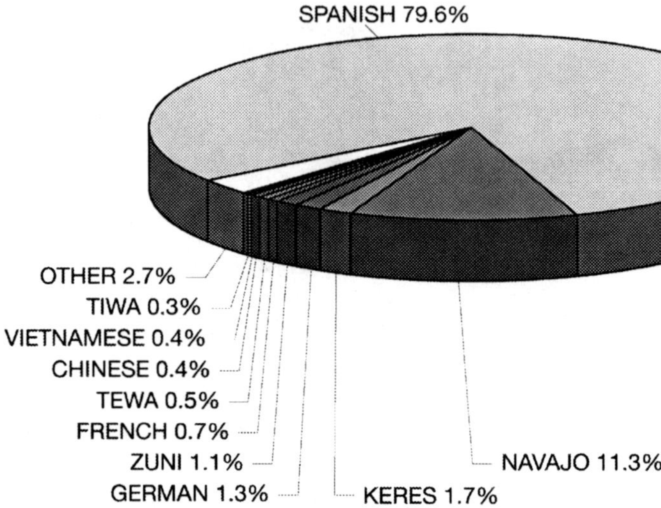

FIGURE 1.5. Pie depiction of the most spoken languages in New Mexico.

phenomenon has been precipitated by the fluid sociopolitical and socioeconomic forces around the world. I am referring to the dissolution of the old Soviet Union, the Bosnia/Croatia conflict, the political instability in the Middle East, Central and South America, and the Caribbean, the economic uncertainty in Japan in the 1990s, etc. The volatility and uncertainty in these regions have resulted in an increase in the immigration patterns from those countries to the United States but also to other parts of the world (Lehrer & Sloan, 2005; Miller, 1991). We are reminded of the frequent illegal boats with human cargoes coming from China, Cuba, Haiti, and the Dominican Republic, with people risking their lives in their attempts to enter the United States in search of a better future.

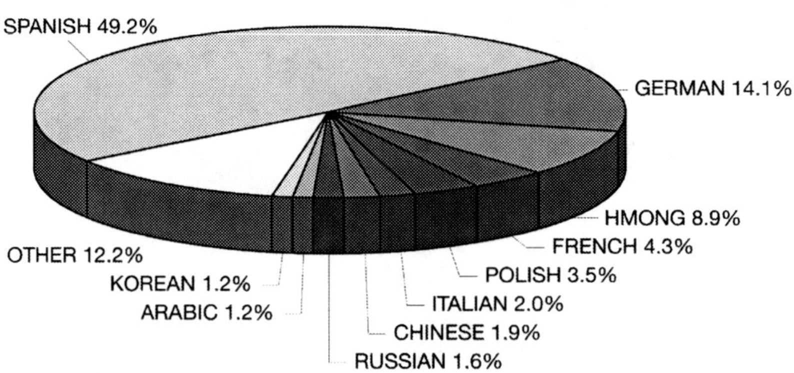

FIGURE 1.6. Pie depiction of the most spoken languages in Wisconsin.

TABLE 1.8. Linguistic groups and the estimated number of people who speak their native language as well as English in the United States, based on the 2000 Census.

Linguistic groups		Proficiency in spoken English	
	Total estimate	Very well	Well
Spanish			
5–17 years	(6,625,553)	4,445,294	1,278,287
18–64 years	(18,519,675)	9,198,012	3,364,412
65 years and +	(1,599,839)	638,245	302,190
Other Indo-European languages			
5–17 years	(1,556,838)	1,206,861	237,170
18–64 years	(6,260,401)	4,177,972	1,293,786
65 years and +	(1,662,431)	991,172	332,815
Asian and Pacific Island languages			
5–17 years	(1,212,386)	839,833	246,477
18–64 years	(5,045,658)	2,451,619	1,465,938
65 years and +	(606,417)	177,356	131,849
Other languages			
5–17 years	(338,961)	269,688	49,073
18–64 years	(1,268,536)	882,207	267,073
65 years and +	(189,102)	114,706	39,277

It is clear from the statistics in Table 1.8 that Spanish-speaking individuals constitute the larger minority language group between the ages 5–17 and 18–64. It also has a large percentage of its members who reported speaking English "very well" or "well"; although, comparatively speaking, individuals speaking Indo-European languages, Asian and Pacific Island languages, and other languages had a larger percentage of its members reporting a good linguistic proficiency in English. It shows the tremendous linguistic acquisition process that takes place among the different linguistic groups while maintaining their original languages. It also shows their commitment to become established in this country. This fact was already evident in the 1976 census that showed that the majority of non-English speakers were born in the US territory. Such a phenomenon clearly affirms bilingualism as a lasting condition in the United States, in spite of the negative movements against it throughout its history.

Fear of Bilingualism?

Thus, we are left with the question as to why the strong negative reaction in some sectors against some of the minority languages and the immigrants? The fact of the matter is that, although the United States and Europe have been confronted with immigration issues over the course of their histories (Miller, 1991), there has not been a concerted effort to address the multiplicity of concerns normally associated with this process, including the challenges associated with multiple languages. At least in the United States, the traditional formula historically used to deal with the challenge caused by immigration of individuals with different cultural, linguistic, and sociopolitical histories is to require from those immigrating full assimilation into the society (the melting pot phenomenon), including requiring the relinquishment of all contact with their languages (Baker, 1993; Bialystok, 2001; Bialystok & Cummins, 2000). This policy of bringing everyone into full compliance with the dominant (linguistic and cultural) society may also have fueled the recent English-only movement in California with Proposition 227 and in Arizona with Proposition 203, referred to earlier, a movement also exacerbated in other states of the Union. What emerges from the argument advanced by those who support such a measure is the tremendous anxiety associated with the presence of another language that is not familiar to the dominant (political) members of our society. It is seen as an infiltration of a linguistic system that threatens the very definition of "being an American" and weakens its institutions' ability to carry out their mission and mandate for the society at large. Lawlessness and chaos are expected to ensue and the United States destroyed as a unified nation with a "Tower of Babel" affliction. Of course, such a fear has not materialized if we consider how the strength of North America comes from its diversity.

Many Western European countries, as we discussed earlier, have also been forced to come to terms with increasing numbers of immigrants seeking asylum, trying to escape poverty, civil unrest, repression, and economic uncertainty. Thus, Europe's normally porous borders are becoming more and more regulated for fear that their societies will be totally overwhelmed and permanently changed by the economic, cultural, and ethnic demands of immigrants. We are reminded of 1991 when boatloads full of Albanians landed in Italy seeking asylum and Italy's decision to return them to Albania (Miller, 1991). Germany, Austria, Switzerland, and France have also been forced to respond to the immigrant issue.

But the European response to this phenomenon has been rather confusing and schizophrenic. In general, most European countries have maintained liberal positions with regard to their immigration policy and hence have tended to welcome immigrants throughout their history to address their specific job/trade needs. One can say that membership in the European Union affirms this policy further in that it allows citizens of European countries to now travel from one country to another in search of better economic conditions.

What is clear is that the increasing concern with terrorism, however, has raised a question about a policy that, although apparently tolerant toward immigrants, has made it difficult for them to become fully integrated into their society (Grosjean, 1982; Miller, 1991), as the recent unrest in France clearly revealed. The discomforting paradox for many European countries is their view that "the immigrant may not be wanted, but they are needed" (Miller, 1991, p. 37). As a result, the host country has not always encouraged assimilation, preferring instead to provide them with separate living arrangements that keep them apart from the rest of society (Grosjean, 1982). Spain's Prime Minister Zapatero is trying to find a different solution but is creating a great deal of controversy in Spain. He proposed an amnesty for those immigrants that have been in the country for more than 5 years. His is a proposal based on an economic decision to ensure collection of taxes from a large population of working people who have been difficult to regulate because of their illegal status.

Thus, with regard to the European solution to the immigrant problem, it is important to consider that the issue is being cast as a socioeconomic and sociopolitical phenomenon while an openness to linguistic diversity is still being maintained. In fact, as we indicated earlier, many European countries are well-known for their bilingual and polyglot communities (Cenoz & Valencia, 1994), specifically, Spain, Switzerland, Belgium, and France. In the Middle East, we can count Israel, South Arabia, and Kuwait. For a pictorial and comprehensive representations of the language distributions around the world see www.ethnologue.com. One can see, for instance, that in France, in addition to the national language, we can also find Basque, Celtic, Germanic, and Romance language families. In Ireland and the United Kingdom, in addition to English, Irish Gaelic and Welsh are spoken. In Portugal, Miranda Do Douro is found, in addition to Portuguese; in Spain, Basque, Aragonese, Catalán–Valencian, Balear, and Galician are found, in addition to Spanish. In Sierra Leone, we find Fuuta Jalon, Bullon So, East Limba, Gola, Susu, and others, in addition to English, as the official language. Finally, in Congo, we find Lingala and Munukutuba, in addition to French.

When we look at some of the countries in South America, we can also see a very rich language distribution. In Argentina, for instance, we find Alacalufan, Araucanian, Austronesian, Quechuan, and Tupi, in addition to the official language, Spanish. And in Venezuela, we find Arawakan, Arutani–Sape, Carib, Chibchan, Salivan, Tupi, and Yanomam, in addition to the official language, Spanish.

Traditional Solution to the Bilingual Problem

There has been a great deal of controversy as to how best to respond to the linguistic needs of immigrants. With regard to educational institutions, the argument put forward by some politicians that the learning of the second language in the young population should be expedited, could be seen, in principle, as having important educational merit. It could be seen as a noble argument in that it seeks to expedite English proficiency among the new immigrants in order to facilitate assimilation into the host educational culture. In this context, those in favor of this argument also lodged a vitriolic assault against bilingual school programs because of the belief that these programs were ineffective in helping the immigrants to become more proficient in English. But what is missing from the argument is the fact that many of these programs were never given the necessary funding to succeed in their mission and hence a true evaluation of effectiveness of these bilingual programs could not be accomplished. The answer to the question of effectiveness is, then, being addressed in the political arena.

Another way used by our society to address the issue of the diverse linguistic community is to marginalize those who, for one reason or another, decide to retain close contacts with their languages and cultures. It is in this way that the various marginal groups were formed in many European cities and cities in the United States (Grosjean, 1982, 1989; Miller, 1991). Although the Hispanic/Latino and Asian individuals have been more clearly identified as part of these marginal and stigmatized groups in the United States, other groups, such as the Polish, Italian, Greek, Hasidic Jew, Haitian, and now the Russian have also formed enclaves in various parts of metropolitan areas where their customs, cultures, religions, and languages are preserved to some degree. Cartographer Guenter Vollath and George Colbert provided a wonderful depiction of these cultural and linguistic distributions in New York City based on the 1980 US census and published in the November 3, 1985, *New York Times* magazine. As discussed earlier, the current 2000 census (US Census, 2000) also shows similar linguistic distribution characteristics throughout the United States and so the general description offered by Lehrer and Sloan (2005).

Unlike the prevalent attitudes previously maintained by individuals with different linguistic histories, bilingual groups are now demanding more understanding from our society in terms of their unique cultural and linguistic needs. They are also demanding more linguistically appropriate programmatic interventions, better teachers, and more study abroad programs that include their countries of origin. They are demanding a stronger emphasis on widening the discussion on the intellectual legacy of thinkers and scholars that historically were not part of the mainstream of the educational system in the United States but were part of the cultural backgrounds of the immigrant groups' cultural and linguistic traditions. Our educational, health, and mental health systems, however, find themselves scrambling to respond to these demands without a full understanding of the unique characteristics of these different linguistic groups. Part of the problem is that our educational system is ill-prepared to address the demands of a bilingual education program. For instance, the problem with teacher's training, material development, community development, poor research on the effect of bilingual education, lack of good curriculum models, and poor quality of instructional materials, although improved, continue to make the viability of bilingual programs questionable (Baker, 1993; Bialystok & Cummins, 2000; Grosjean, 1982).

Current State of Affairs and the Bilingual Phenomenon

Our world is shrinking rapidly and the phenomenon of bilingualism in the United States and other nations is likely to continue growing at the rapid pace witnessed over the past decades. In the United States, Latinos/Hispanics constitute the fastest-growing minority group and is expected to become the largest minority group by the year 2010 (US Census 2000). Immigration from Asia is also rapidly increasing. In addition, the United States is constantly interacting with various countries in Europe, Asia, the Middle East, and Latin America and, although English may be considered one of the diplomatic languages, there is still ample room for misunderstandings and miscommunication without adequate knowledge of the many "faces" of bilingualism.

The September 11 attack on the World Trade Center placed the United States, but also the world at large, once again, in direct relation with individuals and foreign governments whose cultural, linguistic, and belief systems are fundamentally different from ours. The possibility for serious misunderstanding (communicative interference) seems to increase exponentially in relation to the level and extent of differences between and among the different linguistic communities. The events of September 11 propelled the West to actively engage in international political dialogue in which communicative clarity and the ability to decipher important meanings are essential. The need for instruction in languages other than English and for understanding the bilingual, multilingual mind, at least in the academic community and among those involved in international transactions, has never been greater.

That the current world affairs are affecting our language is seen in the introduction of words such as "al-Qaeda al-Sulbah," rather than the translation "the solid base," to refer to specific extremist Muslim terrorist group in the Middle East; "Al-Jihad," a violent and highly secretive organization (*Time*, November 12, 2001); "burka," to refer to "the head-to-toe garment" expected to be worn by the Afghanistan women, especially during the Taliban oppression (*Time*, December 3, 2001); the "Hamas" in Palestine, to refer to that specific terrorist organization in our everyday conversation. This is an interesting development, considering the previous tendency to refer to similar groups by their translated names, such as the "Shining Path," rather than by it original name "Sendero Luminoso," a terrorist group in Perú.

Germany's attempt to deal with the infiltration of English words, such as "laptop," "fit-in," and "event," into the German lexicon was to provide a list of appropriate German lexicon that should be used instead (National Public Radio or NPR, 3/6/02). Thus, the bilingual phenomenon has national and international implications for the United States and the world. And yet, our society's understanding of bilingualism and of individuals with different linguistic histories remains poor.

President George W. Bush had a tough training in the first few months of the first term of his presidency in terms of understanding the importance of international knowledge. His previous preelection position of criticizing the emphasis of the United States' active involvement in world affairs by his predecesor, gave room to his stark realization that the United States will only be able to sustain its position in the world through direct and/or indirect involvement in the world's affairs. This realization now needs to be translated into concrete and sustainable initiatives, such as the establishment of educational/research/political/ economic structures or a "think tank" in the United States whose basic function is to foster and deepen our understanding of other cultures and linguistic societies in the world and in our midst. Specific educational programs should be instituted in our colleges and universities to prepare our next generation of Americans to become more culturally and linguistically sophisticated. It is an inescapable task, especially if the United States is going to effectively fulfill its leadership obligation in the world, which could not be accomplished if only insisting in a primacy of a policy of military involvement.

The Challenge

The understanding of bilingual individuals and their cultural characteristics presents a significant challenge because it involves not only understanding the mechanisms that make bilingualism so unique, but also involves understanding the impact of this process in the whole cognitive and learning process, personality formation, and emotional conditions. In fact, the pervasive quality of language with regard to these processes has motivated psycholinguistic researchers to focus their efforts on the study of the effects of bilingualism (acquisition of two linguistic codes) on processes such as perception, memory, intelligence, learning, and personality formation. There are serious consequences when the issue of bilingualism is not properly considered in education, psychological evaluation, health, and mental health delivery (Albert & Obler, 1978; Bialystok, 2000, 2001; Camacho-Gingerich, 2002, 2004; Cummins, 2001; Fishman, Cooper, & Ma, 1975; Genesee, 2001; Javier, Barroso, & Muñóz, 1993; Javier & Marcos, 1989; Javier, Vazquez & Marcos, 1998). For instance, issues of bilingualism and linguistic diversity have been found to be involved in an increase in diagnoses of learning disability and academic problems in children, as well as in the assessment of emotional disturbances in bilingual children and adults (Alpert & Marcos, 1976; Flanagan, McGrew, & Ortiz, 2000; Javier, 1996; Marcos, 1976). The bilingual mind does appear to function differently than the monolingual mind with regard to memory function, language processing and accessibility of information, and other cognitive and emotional processes (Centeno & Obler, 2001; Hull, 2003; Javier, 1996; Obler, Centeno, & Eng, 1995). Whether such apparent differences are to be construed as reflective of different brain organization has been seriously questioned by Paradis on the basis, among other things, of not clear ways of understanding and explaining contradictory findings on apparently the same linguistic phenomenon (2003, 2004 personal communication).

Recognizing that the changes around the world continue to encourage large numbers of individuals to immigrate to other countries (including to the United States) has forced a change in the ways we educate our children, the treatment and evaluation of these individuals, the way our legal/penal systems need to operate, and how many neighborhoods are now being transformed in their basic characters and becoming more linguistically and culturally diverse. Thus, we thought that our professional and scientific communities in particular, and our society in general, could benefit from a scholarly book about bilingualism and its effect on the cognitive, emotional, and social development of the bilingual individual and hence our decision to prepare this book. This is, indeed, the goal of this book, to fill a void in the professional and scientific community in terms of its understanding of the many ways bilingualism is affecting our society in subtle and direct ways. The book is written for the benefit of scholars, educators, educational and clinical evaluators, clinicians, and students interested in the study of the bilingual phenomenon. The book is also expected to have policy and programmatic implications with regard to education and treatment intervention for this population.

The book will cover issues pertaining to the bilingual mind, emotional development, and the bilingual organization and their role in learning and the evaluation of cognitive and emotional processes. In this context, we have included chapters to address the issue of whether or not there is such a thing as a bilingual mind as well as the issue of how memory develops in bilinguals, because of the implication of these processes in the extent of generalization of learning across languages possible in bilingualism and on the possible impact of the bilingual organization on the whole learning process. A chapter is also dedicated to a discussion of language and emotion and another chapter deals with the problems with translation and interpretation. Another chapter addresses the issues of assessment in the bilingual context with some reference to the impact of environmental substances (such as the effect of lead intoxication) on language development and subsequent scholastic achievement. Finally, a discussion on the future of bilingualism and specific comments on the need to establish more favorable policies on bilingualism that are more reflective of the unique contribution of bilingualism in our society functions as the concluding chapter for this book. It is not meant to be a comprehensive book on bilingualism but rather to function as an invitation to other scholars to engage, in their individual endeavors, in a systematic effort to address issues of bilingualism in all its forms. I hope that you find the book not only informative by enjoyable as well.

2 Is There a Bilingual Mind?

Since the very beginning of the study of human cognitive development, language has been closely associated with almost all aspects of human condition. Many linguistic formulations have repeatedly pointed out the importance of "naming" or the power of "logos" (word) as the process by which "reality" and other "impressions" become organized into units of systems, concepts, or categories. Indeed, the process of naming, which is one of the important aspects of language, transforms the "world of sense impression, which the animals also possess, into a mental world, a world of ideas and meanings" (Cassirer, 1953, p. 28). Once accomplished, the individual is able to transcend the limitation of time and space (Ginsburg & Opper, 1969; Piaget, 1980) and venture into the world of thoughts and mental creations.

We see this transforming process in operation from the very beginning in the lives of children while learning to code their experiences, beginning with an unintelligible, nonsense babbling to a defined utterance. We are reminded of the tremendous joy experienced by parents when hearing the first utterance from their child–"dada," "mom," "baby," "chair," "spoon," "the doggy," "milk." It is quite an awesome experience to observe very young children attempting to communicate even nonverbally and, judging from Figure 2.1, quite effectively. It demonstrates the powerful and ingenious ways the intention to communicate finds expressions even when verbal skills are still at an embryonic stage.

At a later point, more complex sentences are uttered and the child's increasing awareness of complex sentence construction becomes evident. According to Clark (1978), children provide evidence of linguistic awareness at a very early age. First, they are able to repair their own speech, then they are able to correct the utterances of others, and finally they are able to provide an explanation as to why certain sentences are possible and how they should be interpreted (Galambos & Goldin-Meadow, 1990). According to these authors, this ability to verbalize metalinguistic judgments is not accomplished until the age of 6. By age 4, however, children already show sensitivity to linguistic markers in spontaneous repairs of their own speech (Galambos & Goldin-Meadow, 1990; Karmiloff-Smith, 1986). The progressive development of metalinguistic awareness observed in children reflects the increasing sophistication and maturation of brain functioning and the child's enormous capacity for the organization of perception and experiences of various kinds. The development of categories and complex memories are then possible, leading to abstract concept formation. It is then possible for experience to be organized and internalized, to become, later on, a point of reference for the understanding and the processing of future experiences

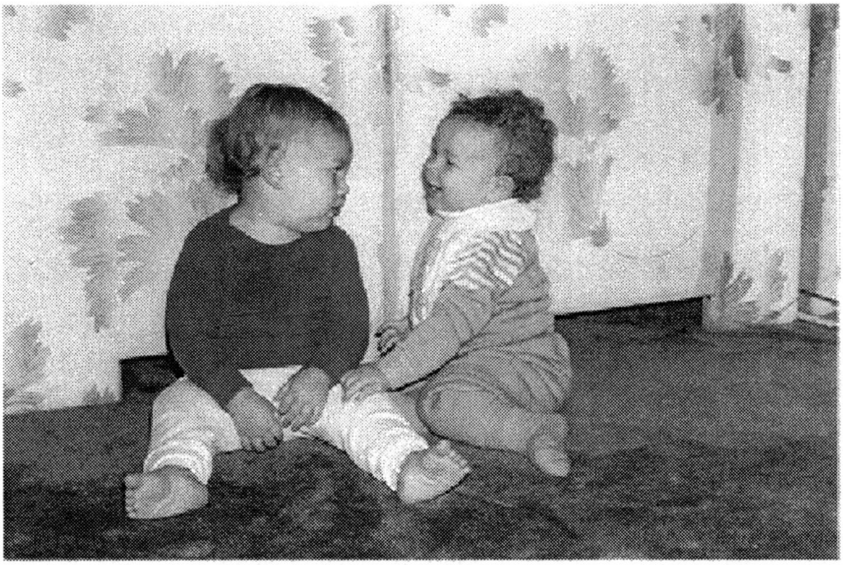

FIGURE 2.1. Two children communicating.

(Mahler, Pine, & Bergman, 1975; Sullivan, 1953). The resulting enduring patterns of organization of these experiences along linguistic dimensions become part of the individual's cognitive structure that then guide the individual's overall function throughout its life.

The importance of this cognitive progression is highlighted, among others, by Piaget (Ginsburg & Opper, 1969; Piaget, 1980, 1995) and Vygotsky (1962) in their theories of cognitive development. According to Vygotsky, for instance, the abstract and symbolic aspects of language (the world of ideas and meanings) make possible the systematization and organization of experiences into categories. It is a verbal mediation position that views language as determining, mediating and thought-producing (Bucci, 1997). Following this line of thinking, Luria and Yudovich (1968) suggested that the most refined expression of the organizing and regulatory effects of language is observed in the way language tends to regulate and categorize the person's behavior. But language also tends to express and reflect the quality of internal organization. It was in this context that assessing the individual's internal cognitive, emotional, and belief patterns became essential in Albert Ellis's work on the individual's belief system (2001) and in Freud's analysis of linguistic contents (1940).

Underlying Luria and Yudovich's formulations is the idea that different categorizations and organizations of the experience may take place with different languages. That is, different cognitive and affective activities may be activated by or may be associated with different languages, depending upon the inherent qualities of these languages. Such formulation found some validation in the works of Whorf (1956), Ervin, (1964), Marcos, Alpert, Urcuyo, and Kesselman (1973) and others. Whorf, for instance, concluded from his comparative study between the Hopi and European languages, including French and English, that the qualities of a language have a determining effect on the way people organize their perception and interpret the world around them. Thus, he discovered that the language of the Hopi processes the idea of "time" and "space" very differently than does the English language. He, then, concluded that these linguistic differences must have a direct bearing on the way the speakers of these languages perceive and interpret the world (Weltanschauung). This is what is known as the "Sapir–Whorf's hypothesis." It is a linguistic determinism but with a dialectical paradigm that suggests that as one thinks so one feels and as one feels so one thinks. Once words have been created to refer to an experience (e.g., time, space, different kinds of snow) these concepts then acquire an organizing power that guides the individual's cognitive process. Thus, the individual is forced to sacrifice whatever variation to the perception that the agreed-upon word is supposed to elicit in order to ensure some level of communication with members of its group. An example of this could be the word "apple" that could mean a green or a red apple, an apple that is small and bitter or juicy and sweet, depending on the individual's experience with apples in the context of his or her cultural and linguistic group membership. Thus, saying that "I just ate a apple," may elicit in the listener only "the apple" of his or her experience, not necessarily the intended message of the speaker, unless additional information is provided.

Studies frequently cited in support of Sapir–Whorf's hypothesis are studies by Ervin (1964), Kolers (1968), and others. Ervin, for instance, observed in her study of thematic apperception test (TAT) cards that her French–English subjects responded differently in the two languages. Responses to the TAT cards in English expressed more achievement themes; responses in French, on the other hand, contained stories with themes involving verbal aggression against peers, autonomy, and withdrawal from others. Similarly, Kolers (1968) and Krapf (1955) observed that different sets of associations, mental representations, memories, and affective responses were elicited in their subjects depending upon the language utilized.

The Bilingual Process in the Context of the Cognitive Development

Because of the crucial role language is assumed to have in cognition and emotion, it is not surprising to see that many psycholinguists are focusing their attention on the effect of bilingualism (the acquisition of two linguistic codes) on processes such as perception, memory, intelligence, learning, and personality formation more and more. Bilingualism is, indeed, a unique phenomenon whose complexity cannot be fully understood by just looking at the way language is developed in general. For bilinguals, two linguistic codes are available at all times to organize and process their perceptions of various kinds (visual, auditory, olfactory, tactile, cutaneous–kinesthetic, see Figure 2.2). So a child who is interacting with its monolingual mother and with whom it learns to communicate and organize its needs (e.g., hunger, physical pain, need for warmth, protection, to have its surrounding explained) and different feelings (e.g., wonderment, feeling of well-being, love, happiness, sadness, discomfort) develops specific linguistic modes of organizing and categorizing these experiences. These organizations and categorizations remain closely connected to the language of the interaction; by that I mean that the unique linguistic (monolingual) characteristics of the family unit where the child grows become encoded in the child's language. What happens, then, when this child now goes to another situation (such as school) where a different language is now utilized for learning and organizing experiences that occur in that context? What happens to these linguistic-specific organizations and categorizations with regard to the whole communication process? Eventually, the child develops ways to organize the different learnings coming from the different sources into its cognitive structure.

What is clear is that the categorization of the experience in the bilingual context and the resulting cognitive structure brings about additional challenges/opportunities to the bilingual individual, not only at the initial stage of language learning but throughout his or her dealing with the world. The understanding of this phenomenon is even further complicated by the fact that not all experiences can be coded linguistically since some of the experiences can remain organized at a prelinguistic or presymbolic level. This is particularly the case for experiences occurring before the symbolic nature of language is developed and acquires the organizing capacity that is possible under a more mature neurological/physiological development. We have seen this phenomenon in operation when a bilingual person is unable to communicate an experience in either language and is left with a general feeling that there is something that cannot be totally and fully expressed in any of the languages. We will come back to this issue when we discuss the role of language in the psychological and emotional development in Chapter 8.

In her recent manuscript "Constructive processes in bilingualism and their cognitive growth effects" Johnson (2000) offers a sophisticated paradigm that seeks to explain the process referred to above in what pertains to the complexity of bilingualism in the context of the whole cognitive process. Following a dialectical–constructive theory, she suggests that the child organizes its experiences in "*knowledge structures*" that follow very specific organization. She distinguishes three basic sorts of knowledge structures that organize the individual's basic cognitive structure: 'infralogical,' 'logological,' and 'linguistic structures.' Infralogical structures are "*particular-experiential structures*" or "*structures of the life-world*" with strong reference to what, I later refer to as, the "first level of experience organization" or experience related to the sensory–motor dimension (Figure 2.2). They are the substance of experience and represent actual objects or things in the environment. According to Johnson, they also include internal representations for distal objects whether they are organized as prototypes, scripts, or schemas. These structures organize the world senses or the concrete physical experiences the child has with its immediate environment. When the "*particular-experiential structures*" (infralogical structures) are

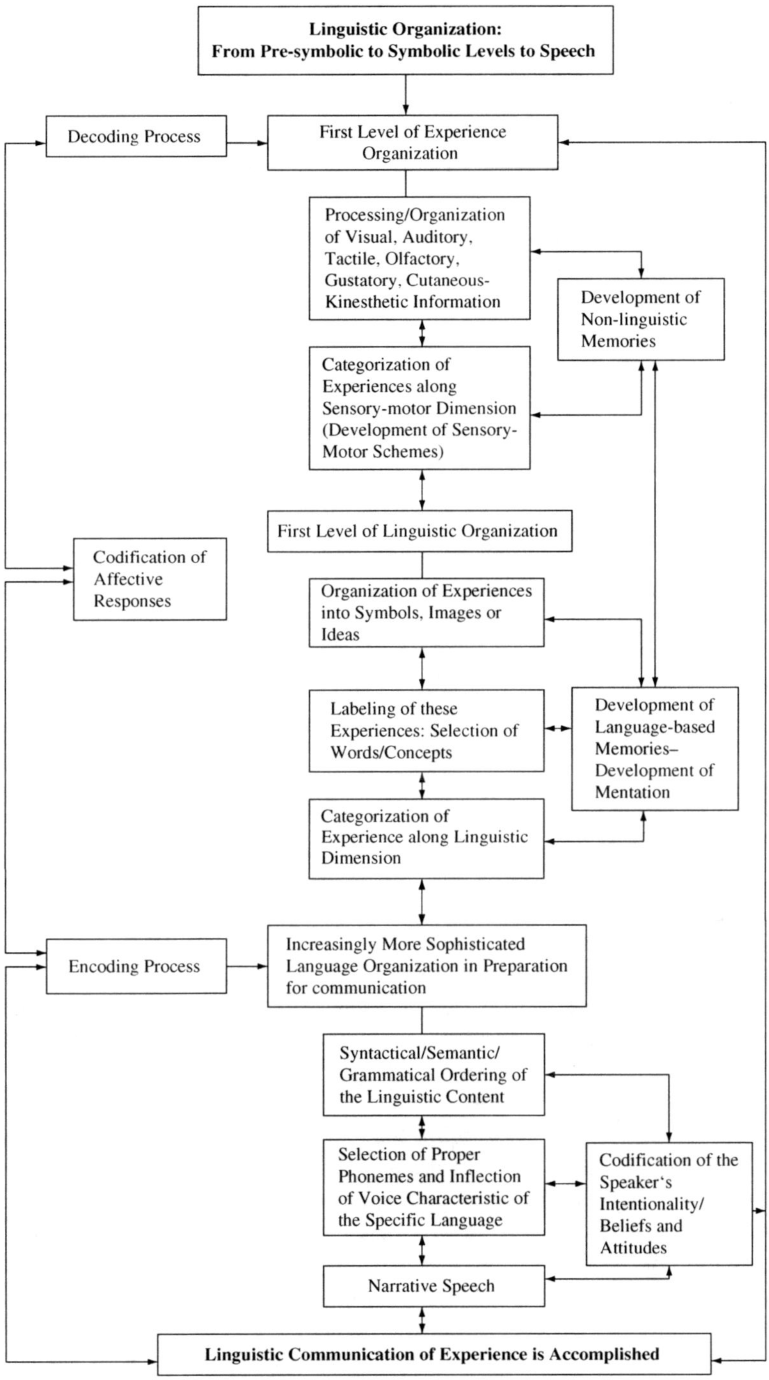

FIGURE 2.2. Process of linguistic organization.

encoded and organized into kinds (or classes, relations, or propositions), logological structures are said to be in place. According to Johnson, logological structures are of a higher order than their infralogical referents; "they are genetic kinds that often represent common characteristics of the infralogical token structures from which they are constructively abstracted" (p. 194). They embody invariances across types of objects or situations and hence they are more abstract structures, higher level or meta-organization, and as such are distinct from the infralogical structures that they can represent. Finally, linguistic structures encode invariances in the linguistic environments (e.g., lexical terms, grammatical relations) and are expected to mediate communication among humans.

According to Johnson, linguistic structures take their meanings from other structures. That is, they denote or symbolize logological structures that, in turn, describe infralogical structures. An important component of this development is that logological structures are not language-specific since, once acquired, "logological knowledge can be language-free ... not reducible to linguistic structures" (p. 194) and can be constructed from the "bottom-up" (by internalized invariances across infralogical structures) or "top-down" (through instruction) through the mediation of language. Linguistic structures do not derive only from logological structures but can derive directly from infralogical structures (such as in the case of signals and many conventional symbols), which the child derives directly from the concrete direct experience with the environment (infralogical structures). An example of this could be the word "mom" that the child could use for organizing experiences related to its interactions with its mother or mothering environment.

The fact that we have a repertoire of experiences that are organized through the logological structures (or genetic-conceptual and hence not language-specific) and others organized through the infralogical structures (or particular-experiential and hence more directly related to the immediate experience) may explain how linguistic situations that are contextualized (e.g., contextualized language skills), or performance produced by structures that are easily cued by concrete features of the situation, are mediated by infralogical structures, while decontextualized information (e.g., decontextualized language skills or of cognitive academic proficiency) are mediated by logological structures. According to Johnson, bilingual information that is organized through and mediated by logological structures can be accessed through either language because it is organized in a metalinguistic manner, while information that is organized and mediated by infralogical structures tends to be language-specific.

According to Johnson (2000), experience with two linguistic systems leads the bilingual child to an early awareness of the arbitrary connection between linguistic forms and meaning. It also facilitates construction of certain kinds of executive structures that guide performance across certain kinds of tasks. These executive structures can be task or control executives and can be logological and infralogical structures. Executives are involved in mental planning and the temporal structuring of mental processing and action across all sorts of tasks.

Task executives monitor the individual's interaction with the environment, while control executives monitor the organismic internal resources or the allocation of cognitive capacities, such as mental attention. Infralogical executives tend to be situation-bound while logological executives are more genetic in nature and hence applicable across contexts.

The importance of Johnson's analysis is that it places linguistic development as part of the development of more comprehensive cognitive structures that provide the individuals with the necessary tools to respond to different challenges. As summarized by Johnson (2000),

> What make sense of experience by means of our infralogical (particular-experiential) structures (i.e., we are always in context). Thus, language as communication has its reference (is validated) at the infralogical level; it is difficult to understand communication that does not make contact with our experience... Developmentally, language starts out having a signalic function... Language also gradually takes on a *symbolic* function, that is, it allows us to entertain the idea of the referent, without making the referent present... Logological structures (the logic of thought) are also symbolic in this sense. (p. 198)

In Figure 2.2 we attempt to provide another view or a schematic representation of this cognitive–linguistic process referred to above but with more emphasis on the linguistic development. Figure 2.2 describes a model of cognitive–linguistic organization from presymbolic to symbolic levels, which finally result in speech production. It is meant to be a dynamic, highly coordinated, efficient, and interdependent model with no reference to the speed with which these functions are normally accomplished. There are multiple loops of interactions assumed to be operative at all times in the communication process and that affect the nature and quality of the final product. It is a synchronic process where the early sensory motor (prelinguistic) stages provide the necessary basis for ultimate developmental accomplishment; that is, the development of mentation and linguistic organization. Many of these functions become automatic over time.

The importance of synchronization of the different aspects of the acquisition of learning (from sensory–motor stages to the development of progressively more complex schemes, to the formation of language proper) was amply discussed by Piaget (Ginsburg & Opper, 1969; Piaget, 1980, 1995) and Locke (1994) who provided specific evidence in this regard. Our effort at this point is only to provide the reader with a visual example, albeit simplistic, of the complexity of the information processing that takes place in each individual in relationship to his or her languages. It implies the linguistic learning that occurs prenatally, described by Locke (1994), and that explains the child's early ability to recognize the mother's voice. According to Locke the child is already involved in the linguistic process in the final trimester of pregnancy when the fetus is capable of hearing the mother's voice. What then follows is a progressive interplay among the different areas that have a direct or indirect impact on the child's final development. This includes the neurological development that makes it possible for the child to process and remember different kinds of stimuli, the maturity of the language sites in the brain, the maturity of the vocal cords and mouth apparatus, the development of the ability to categorize perceptions of various kinds, etc. (Fagen & Prigot, 1993; Luria, 1973, 1981). Thus, at the beginning a child tends to look around its surroundings and eventually begins to babble and repeat sounds made by those around it. At the end, the child learns to say specific words and simple sentences related to its immediate survival (milk, mom, dad, "mom, milk", "my tomy hurts," etc.) with more and more clarity. With the locomotor development (kicking response and the capacity to crawl and then walk), the child develops an array of physical reactions to stimuli in the environment [the kicking response studied by Fagen (1980) and Fagen and his team (1984, 1985, 1990, 2001) in response to different presentation schedules of specific stimuli]. It later starts to venture into other areas that had, up to that point, only been accessible in the context of its interaction with the mother and others who would have carried the child from places to places as they went about their business; and thus begins the process of cognitive/emotional independence (Mahler et al. 1975). It is at this point that the child, although relying, for the most part, on infralogical structures to organize its experience, it also begins to organize its experience in ways that can be stored in memory (object constancy) and categorized at a more abstract mode. This is what Johnson refers to as the beginning of experience organization along the dimension of logological structures. Affects are thus developed in this context and become intimately interconnected with the cognitive development, becoming part of the progressive organization of behavior. This process was amply described by Piaget in his description of the cognitive/affective development of the child (Ginsburg & Opper, 1969; Piaget, 1954, 1995) and Mahler, Pine, and Bergman (1975) in what pertains to the emotional development in the book *The Psychological Birth of the Child.*

The role of language in the organization of experience was also eloquently described by Sullivan (1953) in his description of the nature of the human experience. His description has some similarities to the one provided by Johnson discussed above, although he was more interested in a description of experience in terms of the emotional development and the development of the personality than a cognitive development. According to Sullivan, experiences are organized along three basic dimensions: the prototaxic, parataxic and syntaxic modes (Figure 2.3). Prototaxic refers to an experience that occurs before symbols are

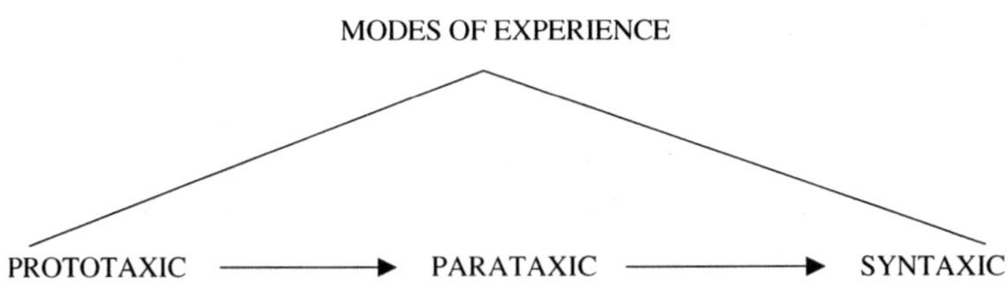

FIGURE 2.3. Sullivan's mode of experience organization.

used; it is the "discrete series of momentary states of the sensitive organism," "it is the rough basis of memory . . . the crudest, the simplest, the earliest, and the most abundant mode of experience" (p. 29). When the child develops symbols as a private and autistic way to communicate these experiences, a parataxic mode is thought to be in place. When these symbols and levels of communication take on a more mature organization that makes possible the easy communication between and among individuals, a syntaxic mode is said to be in place. Thus, a syntaxic mode allows the experience to be communicated to another person. It would be a great mistake to assume that no cognitive organization is in place at the prototaxic or parataxic linguistic organization (Figure 2.3), because it would overlook the complexity of cognitive development prior to the solidification and maturity of the linguistic dimension. In fact, there is evidence of complex thought and learning processes in prelinguistic or prototaxic/parataxic infants (Fagen, 1980; Fagen & Prigot, 1993) and even in adults (Bucci, 1997), as discussed earlier.

In trying to provide further clarification of the complexity of language operation, Friederici (2001) also suggests similar paradigm as proposed by Sullivan but following a more linguistic conceptualization. She suggests that language processing is based on three knowledge sources (semantics, syntax, and phonology, including prosody) that must be activated and well-coordinated in time to guarantee normal language production and comprehension. It is an enormous task. These sources are the essence of the individuals language system and are organized along the procedural (implicit) memory structure, while verbal communication, or pragmatic aspects of the language and metalinguistic knowledge, are organized along declarative (explicit) memory structure (Paradis, 2003). One can then appreciate that the tremendous amount and complexity of timely coordination referred to in the case of a monolingual individuals language processing becomes even more so when more than one language is involved.

No Single Theory can Explain Cognitive Development in a Bilingual Context

The point to be made here is that language processing and the linguistic codification of experience in bilingualism are rather complex and cannot be explained solely following a theory that stresses only one aspect of the linguistic phenomenon. Thus, if we were to follow Chomsky's formulation (1957, 1965), often utilized to explain language development, how are we to apply his conceptualizations to language development in bilingual individuals? Chomsky's emphasis on the innate and universal quality of language with regard to its syntax, which suggests that the individual already comes wired with a capacity for syntactical linguistic organization, leaves us with a number of questions regarding how this capacity influence language development in bilingualism and how other more complex cognitive processes can be explained. Are each of the languages pre-wired in the bilingual individual and what parts of the brain are pre-selected for the operation of the bilingual's two languages? How can Chomsky's formulation explain the findings discussed later in this chapter, that different parts of the brain are involved in language function in bilinguals as a function of when in their development the languages were learned and the level of linguistic proficient acquired? In fact, Chomsky's formulation has been criticized as not comprehensive enough to explain all important aspects of language (Bucci, 1977), and this is particularly the case when referring to bilingualism. Vygotsky's linguistic mediation paradigm (1962) emphasizes, on the other hand, the more dynamic aspects of language. He suggests that language mediates and determines human behavior and all cognitive processes. Mental development is seen as the result of word meanings that come to dominate all human mental processes (Rieber & Wollock, 1997).

In the final analysis, language can only be the product of an interactive and dynamic process combining inherent linguistic and cognitive qualities with the individual's desire to communicate, in the context of the personal and interpersonal realm. Or, as further delineated by Bucci (1997), "communicative language arises from application of general cognitive capacities to the function of communication over vocal and auditory channels" (p. 79). And the fact that we have evidence, in the works of Ervin (1964) and Ervin and Osgood (1954) referred to earlier, that language also tends to mediate perception, confirms the need to maintain a view of language that incorporates these different perspectives.

What make language so powerful are the symbolic complexities that are possible and that eventually result in the transmission of a thought. A thought is a solidification of an intricate process, resulting in the development of an organized schema that encapsulates an experience or set of experiences, an idea or set of ideas, a feeling or set of feelings, etc. According to Bucci (1997), "symbols are entities that refers to other entities and have the capacity to be combined in rule-governed way, so that infinite array of meaningful units can be generated from a finite set of elements" (p. 77). Once the symbols are generated, they function as organizing principles of experience. Thus, images, visual stimuli, and words can then serve as a guiding force for specific experiences (Fagen & Prigot, 1993; Ginsburg & Opper, 1969; Javier & Marcos, 1989).

In the case of bilingual individuals, the symbolic complexities of language become even more powerful. We may be able to visualize the complexity of the bilingual process by imagining a linguistic organization side by side to the one depicted in Figure 2.2. The one depicted in this figure describes a monolingual process. In the bilingual process, we assume that two languages are expected to become involved in the cognitive process, even in the prelinguistic organization level, but more clearly so from the first level of linguistic organization on. We suspect that the extent to which the bilingual's languages will operate more or less independently from one another with regard to these different aspects of language depicted in Figure 2.2 is a function of when and how the two languages are acquired and organized, the level of proficiency in the two languages, and the language function under consideration (Johnson, 2000).

Evidence of the Bilingual Mind?

The confusing and controversial nature of the evidence usually presented in support of the existence of a different and distinct brain organization in bilingual individuals does not allow us to make a definite pronouncement in this regard, leaving us instead with a number of questions in need of more rigorous research paradigms. Paradis (2003), one of the most ardent critics of the existent literature on the subject, finds problems in much of the research literature in this regard at the level of conceptualization, definition of the constructs being studied, and methodology. While recognizing the importance of the need of more rigorous research paradigms, there are data coming from different sources that should be considered in determining the extent to which bilingualism does or does not result in a different linguistic, cognitive, and emotional organization and hence these will be presented at this point.

For instance, the evidence supporting the distinctive characteristics of the bilingual mind continues to mount (Albert & Obler, 1978; Hahne, 2001; Perani, Paulesu, Galles, & associates, 1998). The assumed separateness of the bilingual languages with regard to linguistic organization and processing has found some support in various fronts (Albert & Obler, 1978; Centeno & Obler, 2001; Ervin, 1964; Hahne, 2001; Lambert, 1972; Lambert, Havelka, & Crosby, 1958). In fact, several findings support the view of the distinctive function of the bilingual brain under certain conditions. For instance, Hahne (2001) concluded from a comparison of studies that attempted to decipher the neural substrate in the bilingual languages that the proficiency level in the second language is the most important variable. For low-proficiency participants, different brain areas are recruited for processing the two languages. For the high-proficiency participants, on the other hand, identical neural substrate is recruited.

When looking at semantic processing during reading, Ardal, Donald, Meuter, Muldrew, and Luce (1990), using the "event-related brain potentials" technique or ERPs, which according to Friederici (2001) provides "a temporal resolution in the millisecond domain with a coarse spatial resolution" (p. 238), found that all participants displayed an N400 component. Its latency, however, was shortest in monolinguals and delayed by 40 ms in bilinguals' second language, as compared with their performance in their first language (Hahne, 2001). Hahne (2001) also cited other similar studies with comparable findings, such as the one by Weber-Fox and Neville (1996) that found that all the bilingual groups studied by these authors displayed an N400 effect, but the peak latency was delayed for the participants who acquired the second language after the age of 11. In a study by Hahne and Friedirici (2001 and also summarized in Hahne 2001 manuscript) that assesses semantic and syntactic processing during auditory sentence comprehension in a group of Japanese native speakers who learned German after the age of 18, it was found that the ERPs of the second language learner differed from those of native listeners with regard to the processing of correct sentences. The most remarkable differences were observed for sentences containing phrase structure violations. Specifically, in contrast to native listeners, the bilingual learners showed "neither a modulation of the early anterior negativity nor of the late positivity" (Hahne, 2001, p. 253), suggesting difficulty in sentence processing and integration. Following a different methodology, Hoover (1992) also found different processing strategies in his Spanish/English bilinguals.

Other findings have also emphasized right hemisphere involvement in the case of bilingual in comparison to monolingual (Albert & Obler, 1975, 1978) and differential brain involvement in the bilingual two languages, in keeping with previous findings reported earlier. (Figure 2.4 provides a visual presentation of

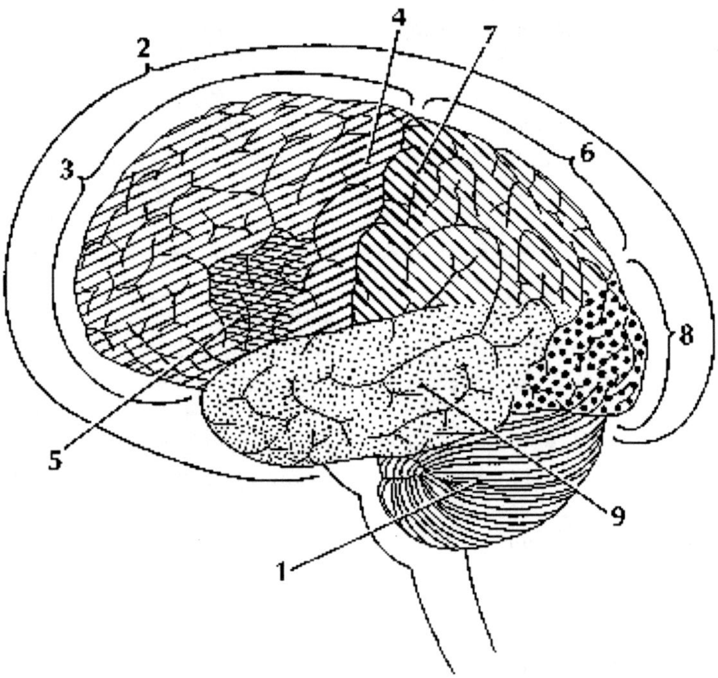

1. Cerebellum
2. Cerebrum
3. Frontal lobes
4. Motor area
5. Broca's area
6. Parietal lobes
7. Sensory areas
8. Occipital lobes
9. Temporal lobes

Published by the National Institute of Neurological Disorders and Stroke. Retrieved from http://www.ninds.nih.gov/disorders/brain_basics/know_your_brain.htm on 11/24/2006

FIGURE 2.4. The architecture of the Brain.

the different parts of the brain that we will be referring to in the context of our discussion. It is a cross-section showing the left part of the brain.) For instance, Ojemann and Whitaker (1978) found that the sites in the center of the speech areas were involved in both languages, while sites in the frontal and parietal cortex were involved in only one of the languages. These authors employed a cortical electrical stimulation technique, placing electrodes in the various parts of the brain for the purpose of assessing the extent of naming disruption in two bilingual subjects.

They found that the right hemisphere was involved in naming in one of the subjects. A differential brain localization was also observed in Chinese–English bilinguals by Rapport, Tan, and Whitaker (1983) in a study discussed by Centeno and Obler (2001). Using cortical electrical stimulation, they observed that language functions were differentially localized along the left perisylvian area. Paradis (1993, 2004) later suggested that these findings are suspicious because the language-specific areas reported only covered the periphery of the language zone and it might be that the stimulation utilized interfered with language only some of the times, with the electrode field falling just outside the language zone at other times. Similarly, it can be said that the findings reported by Albert and Obler (1978), that different aphasic conditions were found in their subjects, were a function of a differential recovery pattern. He explains the different recovery patterns that are observed in aphasic patients as being a function of two kinds of memories that tend to guide language function: declarative and procedural memories. Declarative (explicit) memory structure is more prevalent in second language function and is bilaterally represented. According to Paradis (1993), the fact that declarative memory is more impacted by age and some brain deterioration (such as in Alzheimer's disease) may explain the differential language behavior observed in bilingual individuals in these contexts.

Studies on bilingual memory provide us with important information regarding the question of the bilingual mind. For instance, some studies on memory storage in bilinguals indicate that bilingual memory may be represented by two functionally independent storage and retrieval systems, one for each language (Kolers, 1963; Tulving & Calotta, 1970). Others support an interdependence storage and suggest that all information exists in a single memory storage (Lopez & Young, 1974; Thorson, 1980). A more comprehensive explanation on the way information is stored was offered by Hines (1978). He concluded from his study that "the situation is far more complex that the interdependent or independent models would suggest. Within a given person's memory, information may be stored in both an independent and an interdependent manner, depending on the type of memory representation (e.g., orthographic, phonemic, or semantic) that is being examined....all bilinguals, regardless of the nature of their second language learning experiences, would share a common memory structure with semantic representations being interdependent and orthographic and phonemic representations being independent" (pp. 23–24). Hines even postulated a unitary common memory structure shared by both languages, with semantic representation being interdependent and orthographic and phonemic representations being independent. Again, the conclusion about common versus independent memory systems refers more to the nature of memory structure (declarative vs. procedural) subserving a specific language system/function being studied. As discussed earlier, phonology, morphology, syntax are subserved by procedural memory and isolated words (semantic) are subserved by declarative memory and hence are less focalized in their representation (Paradis, 1994, 2003).

What is clear with regard to studies on the bilingual memory is that the organization of information along a linguistic dimension in a bilingual process appears to be different as compared with a monolingual process. It is experienced as different by the bilingual individual under certain conditions. Thus, the argument put forward by Paradis (1993, 2004) about the two types of memory structures guiding language function in general and the way these structures are reflected in the bilingual individuals as an argument against findings of the apparent brain lateralization and more or less right hemisphere involvement does not completely explain the report of many bilinguals that something is experienced as different when they interact in one or another of their languages (Javier, 1996). Thus, in answering the question as to whether or not there is a bilingual mind, some of the evidence clearly points to the fact that a bilingual person does seem to organize his or her experiences cognitively and emotionally differently in the two languages and that these differences tend to show in obvious and more subtle ways. Because of the centrality of this basic quality of the bilingual experience, we will continue to address this issue more fully in ensuing chapters and, most immediately, in relationship to a discussion on linguistic organization and bilingual memory.

The most powerful evidence in support of the bilingual mind, however, comes from clinical reports of patients who feel that major components of their experiences seem to be language-specific in terms of their ability to retrieve them. Like the patient discussed by Quiñones (2007) who refused to speak her primary language (Spanish) and tried to incorporate an identity that was closer to her ideal image of a successful woman in an English-speaking community. Her style of dress and mannerism, taste of music, and food all changed to be consistent with this acquired identity. She was afraid to speak in Spanish because she did not want to associate with her past and to have to feel the same way she felt when she was emotionally neglected and abandoned by her mother. Thus, her language use was influenced by her need to protect herself from painful memories that she felt were closely associated with Spanish. It is clear that for this patient the two languages provided her with two different alternatives to organize her experience and her personal identity. This is in keeping with the report of adopted children who report not to remember their native language and not to remember anything of their experience associated with that language. Their memory seems to begin with the beginning of the new experience with their adopted families where a new language (second language) was acquired, which is now used to organize and communicate their experiences.

We can tentatively conclude from all these findings that there is some evidence supporting the view that a bilingual individual does tend to process information differently than does the monolingual with regard to different aspects of language processing (semantic and syntactic). The evidence supporting the view that differences in processing in language-specific information found among bilinguals are related to differences in the way a bilingual and a monolingual brain processes information is less clear.

3
The Bilingual Linguistic Organization

If one asks a bilingual individual to relate an experience in one language, it is possible to get different affective responses and more or less elaboration of the experience depending upon the language utilized to communicate such an experience (Javier et al., 1993). The bilingual may feel more or less emotionally connected to the experience being related, resulting in some situations in what Marcos (1976) called "affective distancing." A bilingual may find, for instance, no compulsion to curse in a second language while showing a great deal of propriety in this regard in the first language (mother tongue). Similarly, concepts learned in the second language as part of a schooling may be more accessible in the second language rather than in the first and, in a different context, more proficient language. Part of the reason for such a difference may be found in the work of Weinreich (1974), Ervin and Osgood (1954), Lambert, Havelka, and Crosby (1958), and most recently in my own work (Javier & Marcos, 1989; Javier et al., 1993). According to these authors, bilinguals can develop their languages differently depending upon the mode of acquisition. Some bilinguals are able to develop and maintain two more or less independent linguistic schemes or "coordinate linguistic organization," while others develop a closer interaction between their languages than is the case in coordinate bilingualism or what we refer here as "compound linguistic organization."

The linguistic separateness of coordinate bilinguals and the unique linguistic quality of the compound bilinguals have been repeatedly reported in experimental studies (Jacobovits & Lambert, 1961; Lambert, Havelka, & Crosby, 1958) and aphasiological observations (Albert & Obler, 1978; Centeno & Obler, 2001; Lambert & Fillenbaum, 1959) as evidence of different linguistic organizations in these individuals, or as evidence of the bilingual mind. Lambert and his associates conclude from their findings that coordinate bilinguals tend to exhibit "greater associative independence of translated equivalents" (1958, p. 243) and "less verbal satiation" (or decrease in the meaning of symbols or signs as a result of their repeated presentations) across language than any other group (Jacobovits & Lambert, 1961, p. 579). The assumption is that their performance in these tasks can only be explained in terms of these individuals' ability to maintain separate languages to process information (or what is referred to as the language independence phenomenon). Similarly, observations on aphasic bilinguals and polyglots with a coordinate linguistic organization suggest that their languages tend to become "differently impaired"

(Albert & Obler, 1978; Lambert & Fillembaum, 1959). Differential localization of the two languages has also been cited (Centeno & Obler, 2001).

The unique characteristic of the coordinate–compound dimension will now be discussed from the perspective of the assumed dual linguistic organization and its impact on memory, cognition, and other learning processes. In the context of this discussion, we will discuss in more detail and critically the research evidence from a variety of sources in support of the existence of the bilingual mind, an issue already referred to in Chapter 2. What I want to emphasize at this point again is that the bilingual mind does appear to result in different cognitive and affective organization of the person's experiences. At least, this is reported by many bilingual individuals. To the extent to which this is the case, learning in general can be affected depending upon the language of instruction, the level of the individual's linguistic proficiency, and the nature of his or her linguistic organization. It has even been suggested that bilingualism may encourage emotional splitting and thus the affective components of the individual's experience becoming unavailable in some situations (Greenson, 1950; Javier, 1996; Marcos, 1976).

The Coordinate–Compound Linguistic Organization Controversy

Considerable controversy exists in the literature with regard to the definition and evaluation of the bilingual linguistic organization. One of the most obvious reasons for this controversy is that a bilingual person tends to be unevenly competent in the various aspects of both languages (Macnamara, 1967; Paradis, 1978). Thus, it is deceptively simple to say that a bilingual person is someone who has the ability to use two different languages as "it leaves open several issues that have been a constant source of confusion and lack of clarity in the theoretical and research literature on this topic" (Hornby, 1977, p. 3). Consequently, any description of the bilingual process has to take into account the degree of competence in both comprehension and production in the spoken as well as the written mode of the languages involved (Mackey, 1962). In this manner, distinctions between the monolingual and the bilingual group and among groups of bilinguals can be more readily made. A proper description of the bilingual process must also address the relative independence of the languages and the different language domains (e.g., semantics, syntax, and phonology, including prosody) (Macnamara, 1967).

Comprehension of the bilingual process increased considerably when Weinreich (1974) and Ervin and Osgood (1954) first introduced the concepts of "compound" and "coordinate" bilingualism, from the perspective of language organization, and "subordinate" bilingualism, from the perspective of proficiency. In differentiating the first two categories, they assume that each is the result of acquiring the second language in a specific manner, and that each category represents a radically different representational mediation process in the brain. Each of these categories is unique in that they reflect specific linguistic organizations affecting the overall cognitive and emotional content as well as the extent of accessibility of content in the two languages. Let's take a close look at these categories:

Compound Linguistic System

Ervin and Osgood describe a compound bilingual as a person who tends to process experiences occurring in either of his or her languages within one linguistic-cognitive scheme (Figure 3.1). That is, two sets of linguistic signs (one for each language) come to be associated at the decoding and encoding level with the "same set of representational mediation processes" (Ervin & Osgood, 1954, pp. 139–140). This group is not thought to maintain an independent grammar for its second language as this language is presumed to be "compound to" or dependent on the first language (Diller, 1974). In addition, the meanings (including metaphorical and emotional elements) are assumed to be "constant in both languages" even though two separate systems of coding these meanings are maintained (Ervin & Osgood, 1954).

The above description raises important theoretical questions since it assumes the existence of only one representational mediation process in the brain, suggesting that both languages should be equally available. According to Weinreich (1974), however, this would only be the case in the "true" compound bilingual. Weinreich further states that the compound bilingual "would not function quite as a native speaker of either language since the units of contents of meaning would represent a merging of related but not identical units of contents of both languages" (Paradis, 1978, p. 165).

There is a type of bilingual who also has one linguistic organization (that of his or her native tongue) and whose second language is markedly deficient. Weinreich (1974) and Diebold (1968) refer to this category as "subordinate bilingualism" to distinguish it from "true compound bilingualism." This distinction is not made by Ervin and Osgood, although it seems to be implicit in their description of compound bilingualism. Specifically, Weinreich states that a

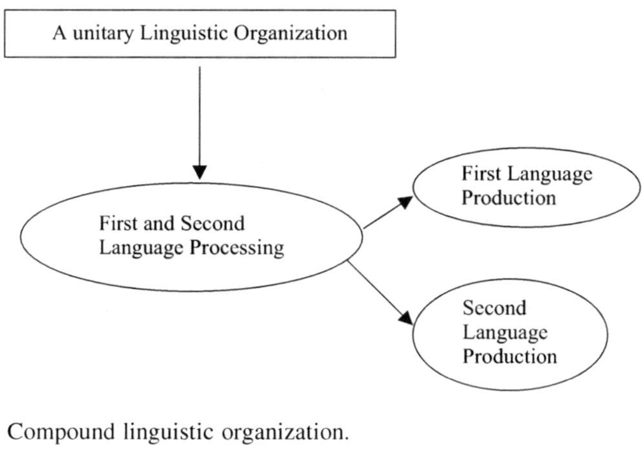

FIGURE 3.1. Compound linguistic organization.

subordinate bilingual is a person who speaks the primary language like a native, but whose use of the second language exhibits a marked deficiency. Weinreich and Diebold indicate that this deficiency exhibited by the subordinate bilingual stems partly from the fact that the second language was acquired through the mediation of the primary one. As a result, the subordinate bilingual tends to use units of expression of the second language to refer to units of meaning of the mother tongue. According to Paradis (1978), this subordination occurs not only at the level of concepts (or meaning units) but also at every level of the linguistic structure, whether morphemic, lexemic, sememic, phonemic, etc.

Marcos et al., (1973) and other investigators have demonstrated the distinctiveness in the behavior of the two groups when they revealed how their subordinate subjects were evaluated as sicker in the second language. Marcos and associates describe the distinct linguistic and paralinguistic elements that made for such a misevaluation and how these elements complicated the psychiatric picture for these patients. Thus, Ervin and Osgood's lack of distinction between the categories of true compound and subordinate bilinguals results in an unfortunate blurring of a significant difference. An example of the importance of this distinctiveness is provided by Paradis (1978) when he states that "in subordinate bilingualism interference is unidirectional" (p. 166); in coordinate–compound bilingualism the interference is expected across the languages.

If we agree that compound and subordinate bilingualism are distinct categories, then different sets of conditions must be responsible for the development of each. As indicated earlier, Ervin and Osgood indirectly describe these two sets of conditions when they discuss the ways in which compound bilingualism develops. They claim that two different sets of learning conditions can contribute to the development of a compound bilingualism.

The first type of learning occurs when the individual learns a foreign language in a school situation through a method stressing vocabulary drill and translation. This condition is assumed to foster association of signs from one language with the signs and their meanings in the other. The second type of learning occurs when "a person grows up in a home environment where both languages are used interchangeably by the same people to refer to the same events and experience" (p. 149). Given the first set of conditions, a subordinate system will eventually be seen rather than a "true" compound, if the speaker's proficiency with the second language remains markedly deficient (Diebold, 1968; Marcos, 1976; Paradis, 1978; Weinreich, 1974).

It should be noted at this point that considerable questions have been raised as to whether compound bilingualism is actually possible. Lambert and Associates (1958), as well as Jacobovits and Lambert (1961), note that the first type of learning situation described by Ervin and Osgood assumes that one linguistic system was already operative at the time the second language was acquired. They claim that this is conducive to the development of a "coordinate system." On a linguistic basis, Diebold (1968) and Diller (1974) question the possibility of developing the "completely unitary semantic structure" assumed in the "true" compound organization, even given Ervin and Osgood's second set of learning conditions. They feel that every aspect of a language is translatable into another language and hence no two languages are completely translatable from one to the other, a phenomenon also eloquently described by Octavio Paz from a literary perspective (1970):

> Ningun texto es enteramente original, porque el lenguaje mismo, en su esencia, es ya una traducción; primero, del mundo no-verbal y, despues, porque cada signo y cada frase es la traducción de otro signo y de otra frase.... Cada traducción es, hasta cierto punto, una invención y así constituye un texto único. (p. 9)

At the risk of violating Octavio Paz's original thought, an approximate translation is as follows:

> No text is entirely original because language itself, in essence, is already a translation, first of the non-verbal world and then because each symbol and phrase is the translation of another symbol and phrase... Each translation is to some extent, an invention and hence constitutes a unique text.

Even under the best of circumstances, as presented by closely related languages, such as Spanish and Italian, there are lexico-semantic-grammatical limitations as well as infralinguistic limitations that make literal translations impossible. At the lexical level, for instance, the English pronoun "you" has two possible translations in Spanish: *tu* (intimate) and *usted* (formal). Similarly, the Greek word *kalos* can be translated "beautiful," "honorable," or "fine," three different English meanings. At the phonemic level, the English sounds /st/ and /sp/ as in "street" and "speak" cannot be found in Spanish and the English sound / ⊖ / like in *"then"* does not exist in Hungarian (Makkai, 1978, p. 51).

This line of reasoning and numerous experimental observations lead Lambert to conceive bilingualism along a continuum. He states that any particular bilingual will develop a compound relation between his or her languages for certain of his or her experiences and a coordinate relation for other experiences (Lambert, 1972, p. 301). Thus, he concludes from he or she experiments that the compound bilingual tends to develop a more or less unitary semantic structure because of the way his or her learns the two languages (Lambert, 1955; Lambert et al., 1958).

Coordinate Linguistic System

As we indicated earlier, a coordinate linguistic system is characteristic of a person who learns a second language independently and in different contexts, as for example exclusively outside the home, or at some later post-infancy period. It is also characterized of someone whose parents used two different languages consistently, as a matter of course, to communicate. In this situation, such an individual will develop two separate sets of linguistic signs, responses, and representational mediation processes (Ervin & Osgood, 1954; Lambert et al., 1958; Marcos, 1976; Paradis, 1978). Presumably, these bilinguals tend to make

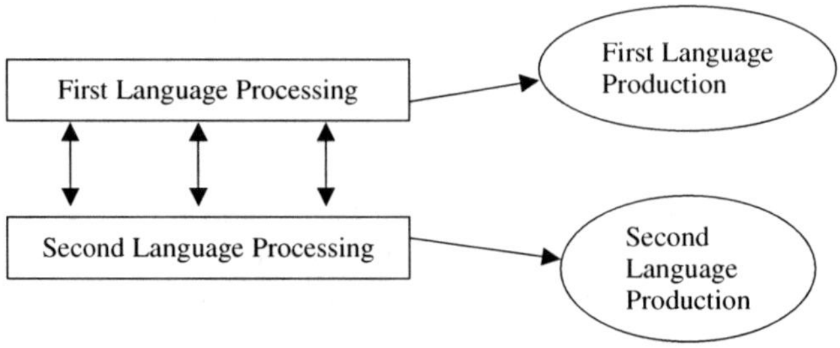

FIGURE 3.2. Coordinate linguistic organization.

minimal or no use of translations (Ervin & Osgood, 1954; Lambert et al., 1958). This group has been considered the "truly" bilingual. This is because they tend to speak both languages well and with minimal interference (Brooks, 1964; Diller, 1974). (Figure 3.2)

It has been observed that if the second language is learned after puberty it is more likely to achieve a relatively independent status (Schnitzer, 1978). Neurological studies (Penfield & Roberts, 1959; Schnitzer, 1978) explained this in terms of brain plasticity that gradually decreases after infancy. An example of this lack of plasticity is the increased presence of foreign accents observed in individuals who acquire their second language in adulthood (Lenneberg, 1976, pp. 180–181). Accent, however, is not the most important element of learning a new language. In fact, accent notwithstanding, Diller (1981) found adults to be much more proficient and faster than 9-year-olds in learning a second language. Similarly, Snow (1981) found that her adult subjects tended to use more efficient information processes and more elaborate language-syntactic processes than her younger subjects. Furthermore, it can be argued that the adult lack of plasticity creates the proper condition for the development of a coordinate linguistic organization. The fact that the brain is already less flexible makes it less likely for the languages to become compounded in the same part of the brain.

The Language Independence Phenomenon

The observed distinctiveness of the coordinate bilingual's languages in terms of perception, learning, memory, emotion, and other experiences is referred to in the literature as the "language independence phenomenon" (Javier, 1996; Marcos, 1976; Marcos & Alpert, 1976). This phenomenon suggests that experiences and memories are stored and mediated separately by each language. Utilizing a group of bilinguals with a coordinate linguistic organization may then provide us with a unique experimental condition that may allow us to evaluate processes such as perception, learning, memory, and emotion as they are related and/or unrelated to linguistic behaviors in a bilingual context. A group of coordinate bilinguals can be conditioned, for instance, to a task involving perception, memory, learning and other aspects of cognition in one language and the effects in the other language can then be assessed.

In a study involving stress and linguistic conditioning we, indeed, attempted to assess the linguistic behavior of a group of coordinate bilinguals in what pertains to the assumed separation of the languages (Javier & Marcos, 1989). Stress has already been found to affect the linguistic behavior of monolinguals (Bridger, 1970; Pope, Blass, Siegman, & Raher, 1970). Pope and associates, for instance, were able to measure anxiety and depression experimentally from the expressive aspects of the subjects' speech (e.g., speech rate, articulation rate, silence quotient, ah ratio, speech disturbance ratio). He found that anxiety and depression had a direct bearing on the linguistic behavior of his monolingual subjects, affecting its production. Similarly, Bridger found that stress or strong emotion (operationally defined by two levels of electric shocks) produced a relative increase in phonemic as compared to semantic generalization. The mild electric shock intensity produced greater semantic than phonemic generalization. The opposite was observed in the case of the strong electric shock intensity. He interpreted this tendency toward phonemic generalization observed in the strong electric shock group as a manifestation of a primitivization of the cognitive functioning of these subjects. This is the case because the normal cognitive progression calls for the individual to move from a phonemic to a semantic linguistic organization of his or her experience as the cognitive process becomes more developmentally mature and more sophisticated.

Similar findings of linguistic primitivization were found in our own study with bilinguals (Javier & Alpert, 1986; Javier & Marcos, 1989), following Bridger's paradigm. Additionally, linguistic switching was observed as well under conditions of stress. The interesting finding was, however, that only under the milder condition of stress a more clear cross-linguistic generalization (more code-switching) was found. In the case of the more intense condition, less code-switching was observed. We concluded in this regard that when a subject is confronted with too disorganizing an experience (an experience eliciting too strong an emotional reaction), the normal process of language organization is disturbed resulting in a primitivization in the cognitive process. This suggests that there is an optimal level of affect in the individual that is conducive to learning and the transfer of information from one language to another. Beyond that critical level, learning and the cross-linguistic generalization of information are deleteriously affected.

The importance of these findings is in lending support to seminal works from a number of authors who demonstrated how stressful and anxiety-provoking experiences tended to stimulate linguistic shifting among bilinguals (Kraph, 1955; Stengel, 1939). Linguistic shifting or "code-switching" (Redlinger, 1976; Weinreich, 1974) refers to conditions in which two linguistic systems, while remaining separate, are brought into contact. Thus, the code-switching phenomenon presumes the existence of the language independence phenomenon.

Psychological/Psychoanalytic Observation

A number of psychoanalytic observations, experimental studies, and aphasiological observations have often been introduced as evidence of the existence of the language independence phenomenon. As referred to earlier, Buxbaum (1949), Greenson (1950), Stengel (1939), Kraph (1955), and others independently noted the remarkable distinctiveness in their bilingual patients' responses in the therapeutic situation, depending upon the language of the treatment (Javier, 1996; Perez-Foster, 1996). They observed that different sets of associations, mental representations, and affective responses were elicited in each language. For instance, Greenson reported the case of a bilingual patient who described herself as a "scared dirty child" in German and as a "nervous refined woman" in English (p. 19), suggesting two different self-definitions. Similarly, Buxbaum (1949) described the case of another bilingual patient who verbalized one stream of associations to the word "sausage" in English and another stream of association to its equivalent in German *blutwurst* (pp. 282–283).

In analyzing the relationship between the linguistic behavior of these patients and their intrapsychic conflicts, these authors observed that their patients would utilize their second (acquired) language during analysis to avoid the emergence of deeply seated infantile conflicts. Thus, primitive conflictual material would remain unavailable for exploration as it remained independent of the language system in which the treatment was conducted. The German woman in treatment with Buxbaum referred to above, for instance, refused to speak in German because this language was associated with memories of a "forbidden infantile curiosity and a guilty sexual relationship" (p. 283). Similarly, Greenson's German woman patient refused at times to speak in German, claiming', "I have the feeling that talking in German I have to remember something I want to forget." She also felt that obscene words were "much easier to say and were much cleaner in English." "A chamber-pot becomes alive if you say *Natchttopf.* It is ugly, disgusting, and smells bad. In English a chamber-pot is much cleaner" (p. 19). Similar cases were reported by Kraph (1955) who concluded that "the common denominator of the motivations that underlie the choice of languages in polyglot psychoanalysis is, in general, a tendency to avoid anxiety" (p. 356).

In examining the language experience of these patients, it appears that they learned the second language in geographical and cultural settings different from those in which they learned their first language. Ervin and Osgood (1954) claim that this condition fosters the functional separation of the two languages and hence the functional independence of the languages.

Psycholinguistic Studies

Following Ervin and Osgood's specifications of coordinate and compound bilingualism, Lambert et al. (1958) classified bilinguals as having learned their languages in either "separated" or "fused" contexts. They used a brief language questionnaire that included questions as to "how", "when", and "where" the languages were acquired. The separated acquisition group included subjects who had acquired their languages in one of three possible manners:

1. Those who learned one language exclusively in the home while the other was learned exclusively outside the home
2. Those who were raised in homes where one parent consistently used one language and the other parent consistently used a different language
3. Those who acquired each language in a different national or cultural setting ("bicultural" group).

From the point of view of linguistic organization, the separated acquisition group is referred to as the coordinate bilingual group.

The fused acquisition context group included subjects who either used both languages interchangeably inside and outside the home or acquired their second language in a school system stressing vocabulary drill and translation, with the first language used as the medium of instruction. From the point of view of linguistic organization, this group is referred to as the compound bilingual group.

Both of these groups were subjected first to a test of "semantic differential" and then to a test of "associative independence." The first of these tests, originally developed by Osgood (1952), asks the subjects to rate four common English concepts (e.g., house, drink, poor, me) and their translations in French along a series of seven-point scales, each representing a bipolar dimension (such as "fast–slow"). The associative independence test was designed using the old retroactive inhibition technique. That is, each subject learned a list of 20 commonly occurring English words by the anticipation method; they were then asked to learn another list of 20 three-letter nonsense words. Finally, they were re-presented with the original list of English words and their retention of the original list was measured. Subsequently, the subjects were asked to learn a second list of 20 English words but this time followed by a list of their exact translations in French instead of the nonsense list.

They found that bilinguals who acquired their languages in separated contexts (coordinate bilinguals), especially those with bicultural experience, showed significantly less interference from the list of translation equivalents than did those who acquired their two languages in fused contexts (compound bilinguals). Similarly, this group demonstrated significantly greater difference in meanings of translated equivalents than did the fused acquisition group. The results also showed that the separated acquisition group demonstrated more associative independence of translation equivalents than those with experience in fused contexts. Indeed, this latter group clearly benefited from the interpolated French list.

Similar results were obtained by Jacobovits and Lambert (1961) in a study of semantic satiation among bilinguals of the same categories as in the previous study. In this experiment, subjects were asked to rapidly repeat a word aloud for 15 seconds and then the amount of change in meaning (or semantic satiation) was determined. Semantic satiation was defined as the "decrease in meaning of a linguistic symbol or sign as a result of its continued presentation" (p. 579). The measurement of this variable was accomplished by comparing the intensity of the rating of words on a semantic differential scale with the intensity rating of the same words prior to the repetition period. Again, the findings showed that coordinate bilinguals demonstrated less tendency for cross-language satiation in meaning than did compound bilinguals.

Paradis (1983) later argued, after reviewing Lambert and Fillenbaum's data that were not presented in the published paper (1959), that there were problems with the proper categorization of subjects along the coordinate–compound paradigm, particularly in the case of the compound group.

The importance of contextual linguistic learning in fostering the functional independence of the languages is further highlighted by Ervin (1964) in her study with TAT, referred to earlier. She obtained a sharp difference in the response to the TAT in a group of French–English bilinguals who were raised in France and learned English when they migrated to the United States later in life. Her subjects verbalized achievement themes more frequently in English TAT stories than in French stories. Themes involving autonomy or withdrawal from others were more common in the French stories. She attributed these results to differences in the behavioral norms of the French and English cultures that are then transmitted through the mediation of language. According to her, French culture does not seem to stress achievement in women. It appears, however, that French culture stresses silent withdrawal as a mode of aggression and emphasizes skills in oral argument, as opposed to physical aggression. Thus, "it is possible that a shift in language is associated with a shift in social roles and emotional attitudes" (p. 506).

Similar results were obtained by Findling (1969) in his study of charactero-logical traits, such as "Need for affiliation" and "Future orientation," in a group of Spanish–English bilinguals. Need for affiliation is defined by the author as the individual's concern to establish, maintain, and restore positive relationships with others. On the other hand, future orientation is defined as the extent to which a person's preoccupation with events that may or may not happen precludes concern with things and events that have already taken place. The results indicate that both of these traits were significantly stronger in English than in Spanish.

Tulving and Calotta's (1970) study of free recall among polyglots proficient in English, French, and Spanish is also often cited as evidence of the language independence phenomenon (Albert & Obler, 1978; McCormack, 1977). These authors visually presented to their subjects unilingual, bilingual, and trilingual lists and instructed them to recall each list orally at its conclusion. Their findings indicate that recall is best from unilingual lists, next best from bilingual lists, and poorest from trilingual lists. These authors interpret poorest recall from the multilingual lists as reflecting an impairment in the organization of words across language boundaries. They suggest, in particular, that the impaired performance in bilingual and trilingual lists resulted not from impaired storage but from impaired accessibility due to the difficulty in forming high-level organizational units from members of the lists. Thus, the independence between the several lexical systems is assumed.

A similar experimental paradigm is utilized by Macnamara and Kushnir (1971) to investigate the bilingual's capacity to interpret linguistically mixed passages. Their English–French bilingual subjects were presented with a unilingual passage and passages with one, two, or three switches. They found that their subjects responded (true or false) fastest to material presented unilingually in their strong language, next fastest to material presented unilingually in the weaker language and next to material containing two switches. The response was lowest for materials containing three language switches. They concluded that "English and French formed psychologically distinct systems" for their subjects (p. 485).

Neurological Evidence

The above studies lead to the conclusion that the languages of the proficient bilinguals tend to be maintained as functionally separate from one another. This is particularly true for those bilinguals who have learned their languages in distinct contexts and have utilized them in settings that encourage their functional separation. Thus, a coordinate linguistic organization is developed. When bilinguals learn their languages in fused acquisition contexts, they develop a compound linguistic organization that is characterized by the functional dependency of the languages on one another.

A basic assumption of this way of conceptualizing bilingualism is that the different learning contexts that result in a functional organization of the languages along the coordinate–compound dimension also result in a comparable linguistic development at the neurological level (Ervin & Osgood, 1954). Thus, neurological damage affecting a speech area (a condition known as aphasia) in a bilingual individual is expected to have a differential effect on his or her two languages. However, the findings reported in this regard are confusing and contradictory, depending on the aspect of the language system under consideration (Paradis, 2003).

Several of the early observations on the subject reveal that, in fact, damage to the speech area of bilingual and polyglot individuals does result in a differential impairment of their languages. It was reported, for instance, that an aphasic condition in bilingual patients resulted in the partial or complete loss of the most recently acquired languages (Ribot, 1882), or in the partial or complete loss of the language least utilized immediately prior to the aphasic condition (Halpern, 1941; Pitres, 1895). The former condition is interpreted in terms of the "rule of Ribot," which states that linguistic habits acquired early in life are more resistant to aphasic damage than those acquired subsequently. The latter is interpreted in terms of the "rule of Pitres," which states that the language most used immediately before the aphasic insult will be the first to recover (Lambert & Fillenbaum, 1959, p. 28). According to Centeno and Obler (2001), Pitres' model has been more successful in explaining linguistic recovery than has Ribot's.

According to Paradis (2004), Pitres' rule seems to apply more to younger patients while Ribot's rule to older patients. In this context, it is expected that older aphasic patients will have greater difficulty with their later-learned language than will younger aphasic patients, since declarative memory (expected to subserve the second language) is more affected than procedural memory by aging. Paradis used Obler and Albert's (1977) analysis of previous reports to support his contention. Obler and Albert found that elderly aphasics did not, in fact, recover their second most familiar language better. That is, elderly aphasic patients tended to have more difficulty with their second language, rather than be affected by the Ribot's rule of regression (where the oldest acquisitions are the most stable and most resistant to morbid dissolution).

Other cases have been reported in which the aphasic damage was found to be limited to the switching mechanism of the languages. Goldstein (1948), for instance, reported the case of a Swedish woman who would shift from English to Swedish for more emotional statements but who could not translate from either language upon command. Similarly, L'Hermitte, Hecaen, Dubois, Culioti, and Tabouret-Keller (1966, cited by Albert & Obler, 1978) reported the case of a 46-year-old right-handed English businessman who lived in France for about 10 years. An oblation of an anterior left temporal lobe glioma resulted in a sensory aphasia characterized by a peculiar influence of his English on his French in both oral and written production.

The impairment of the switching mechanism is frequently utilized as an argument in favor of the existence of two separate linguistic systems as "it is difficult to conceive of a switch without assuming that there are two separate systems between which the switch operates" (Albert & Obler, 1978, p. 232). According to Obler, Centeno, and Eng (1995), however, there is no evidence supporting the existence of a specific anatomical location of a switch mechanism in the brain. This is the case because for the few articles reporting deficits of the switching mechanism, the lesions have not occurred in the same or overlapping areas. They are more comfortable endorsing a monitoring mechanism that is quite diffusely organized in the brain.

Some polyglots have also been reported to display different types of aphasic syndromes. A case in point is that of a right-handed Hungarian-born polyglot woman with knowledge of French, English, and Hebrew in addition to her native language. After a partial oblation of a large left posterio-temporal glioma, she was found to display a Wernicke's aphasic condition in English and a Broca's aphasic condition in Hebrew (Albert & Obler, 1975). Similar cases of different aphasic syndromes were reported by Wechsler (1977), Lyman, Kwan, and Chao (1938) and by Nair and Virmani (1973). Wernicke's aphasia refers to the condition in which the capacity for a fluent, paraphasic speech is maintained but in which the capacity for comprehension is impaired. Broca's aphasia, on the other hand, refers to the condition in which the capacity to comprehend speech is maintained but in which the capacity to produce spontaneous speech is impaired (Gardner, 1976).

Paradis (2004) took issue with these apparently different aphasic conditions reported, suggesting that the problem was more a function of misdiagnosis. According to this author, to begin with, it is difficult to ascertain the accurate extent to which premorbid proficiency in all the languages existed. Under the best of circumstances, it is rare to find equivalent fluency or comprehension in the several languages of the healthy polyglots. Thus, the differential performance exhibited post brain trauma may be only a reflection of the premorbid state of affairs. In the case reported by Albert and Obler (1975), Paradis' contention is that it is a case of differential recovery pattern, rather than differential aphasia, and that the patient exhibited symptoms of Broca's aphasia in both languages.

Albert and Obler's (1978) more comprehensive analysis of previously reported evidence of language-specific impact of brain trauma attempted to throw more light on the question of the differential language-specific brain organization. They examined 108 cases, 70 of which had known lesion information. They observed that 7 of these cases had a right hemisphere lesion, 53 cases had left hemisphere lesion, and 10 cases had bilateral lesion. Of the seven right hemisphere cases, there were three left-handers, three right-handers, and for one the premorbid handedness was unknown. They found that younger polyglots were more likely to have aphasia from right hemisphere lesions than were younger monolinguals while the oldest group evidenced no exclusively right-sided lesions. These authors concluded that "younger polyglots are more likely to have aphasia from right hemispheric lesions than are younger monolinguals. This would imply that a greater percentage of polyglots than monolinguals have some right hemispheric representation of language" (p. 143).

Albert and Obler (1978) also examined the earlier stated assumption that the linguistic organization of coordinate bilinguals at the neurological level is expected to differ from a compound linguistic organization. These authors expected that their coordinate bilinguals would show more selective deficits as a consequence of brain damage than would compound bilinguals, who are expected to show a more generalized linguistic effect after brain damage. Contrary to this expectation, however, they found that compounds (81%) were more likely than coordinates (71%) to show a discrepant (differential) aphasic picture and that more coordinates (28%) than compounds (18%) showed parallel recovery (both languages recovered at the same time).

This issue was also examined by Lambert and Fillenbaum (1959) who compared 14 cases of polyglot aphasics from Europe reported by Leischner (1948) with 14 cases of their own that they collected in Montreal, and then with the cases reported by Pitres (1895). These authors reasoned that most of the cases reported by Pitres and those obtained in Montreal were likely to have developed a compound linguistic organization since these polyglots and bilinguals seemed to have learned and utilized their languages in the same geographical and social contexts. For the European patients, however, the second language was assumed to be typically learned in a context distinctly separate from the first, thus encouraging a coordinate linguistic organization.

They found that, contrary to Albert and Obler's findings, "the Montreal cases typically show a generalized disorder affecting both languages, while the European cases typically show a more language-specific disorder following aphasia" (Lambert, 1972, p. 76). That is, patients whose linguistic histories suggest that they would essentially have a compound organization showed equal deficit in both languages whereas those patients who would generally have a coordinate linguistic organization because of the separate ways they learned the second language suffered a more language-specific disorder.

In order to understand the apparently discrepant findings discussed above, it is important to appreciate the nature of the difficulties that these authors had in establishing the correct bilingual groups to which their subjects belonged. Many of these subjects lacked sufficient premorbid linguistic history and thus the decision to judge them as coordinates or compounds could not be clearly delineated. This is especially true in many of the cases reviewed by Albert and Obler. Specifically, these authors tended to categorize as compound many cases that might elsewhere be categorized as coordinates. For example, a case reported by Charlton (1964) of a 40-year-old woman who learned English as her second language when she was 10 years old and the case reported by L'Hermitte et al. (1966) of a 48-year-old man who learned French as a second language when he was 8 years old were both categorized by Albert and Obler as fitting the description of compound bilingualism. It appears, however, that in both of these cases one language was already operative when the second one was acquired; thus, the development of a coordinate linguistic organization rather than a compound one is suspected.

Albert and Obler's failure to obtain significant differences between compound and coordinate bilingual groups with regard to the kind and extent of linguistic deficit after brain damage may be attributable to their difficulties in categorization. Consequently, their percentage of compound bilinguals showing a discrepant (differential) aphasic picture may very well be lower than 81%, while their percentage of coordinate bilinguals showing a discrepant aphasic picture may be higher than 71%.

Conclusion

Although the neurological evidence of the language-specific brain organization cannot be considered as conclusive because of the problems with these types of data, other data coming from some psycholinguistic and observational studies are more promising. We can at least conclude that the bilingual's languages do offer the individual unique opportunities to organize his or her experience differently and are guided by the language independence phenomenon. It is clear, however, that more systematic studies on the subjects are called for before a more conclusive statement is made in this regard. It is true that the coordinate–compound paradigm has offered a good way to organize different linguistic groups for the purpose of control research; the literature, however, remains confusing in terms of how the subjects are categorized, how the stimuli being studied are defined, the level of validity of method utilized, etc.

This is in keeping with the call for more systematic and careful line of investigations that Paradis made in his recent publication (2003) with regard to brain lateralization in bilinguals. According to Paradis (2003, p. 446), "before we can say anything about laterality in bilingual speakers on the basis of dichotic, visual hemifield tachistoscopic, verbal–manual procedures and other experimental methods, these methods must be shown to be valid." By which he means that one should:

1. Define clearly what is alleged to be or not to be asymmetrically represented.
2. Demonstrate that the stimuli used in the specific experiment are actually tapping into language system, as defined.
3. Come up with a rationale for why there should or should not be any difference in hemispheric asymmetry between unilinguals and any subtype of bilingual speakers.
4. And finally, demonstrate that the instrument utilized truly measures degrees of cerebral laterality.

4
Language Switching As a Communication

It is quite amazing and fascinating to observe bilingual individuals changing languages in the middle of a conversation with other bilinguals as they go from one topic to another, or as they interact with monolingual members from any of their languages. And this is done automatically in a more or less conscious state. Being able to change languages when the situation calls for it is, indeed, one of the most fundamental qualities of bilingualism. It involves not only the capacity to maintain languages separately but also the ability to bring them into contact when the situation calls for it. This process is referred to as "code-switching phenomenon" (Javier & Marcos, 1989; Redlinger, 1976; Weinreich, 1974). It is the process by which the bilingual individual manages "to set aside a whole integrated linguistic system while functioning with a second one and, moments later, if the situation calls for it, switch the process, activating the previously inactive system and setting aside the previously active one" (Lambert, 1972, p. 300). Thus, the phenomenon assumes the relative independence of the languages since the organizational principles and grammatical structures and phonemic elements have to be maintained, under the best of circumstances, nearly intact in the languages involved, in accordance with the norms of the monolingual communities for each of the languages (Shaffer, 1978). That is, it requires a certain level of functional proficiency in each of the languages, which then allows the interplay between the languages while adhering to the grammatical, syntactical, and phonetic rules of each of the languages involved.

Again, this process is highly automatic; those involved in the switching engage in a highly sophisticated process of assessing all the cues in the environment where the interaction is taking place to determine appropriateness and accuracy. In the final analysis, the process is guided by the intentionality of the speaker to communicate specific content, at a specific time, for specific effect, albeit not always consciously clear to those involved.

As discussed in Chapter 3, some investigators have tried to explain the operation of this process in terms of the neurologically based switching mechanism (Leischner, 1948; Penfield & Roberts, 1959) or a monitoring mechanism diffusely organized in the brain (Obler, Centeno, & Eng, 1995). Others have tried to describe the behaviors and psychological characteristics of this mechanism and have tried to identify conditions under which switching tends to occur (Lispki, 1978; Macnamara & Kushnir, 1971; Wakefield, Bradley, Byong-Hee, Yom, & Doughtie, 1975). Of the two ways of approaching the issue, only the latter has been useful, because we have not been possible to detect a neurological mechanism directly responsible for language switching. So, for instance, aphasiological observations by Goldstein (1948) and L'Hermitte et al., (1966) reveal that this mechanism was impaired in some of their aphasic patients. But it is not yet known, however, what part of the brain is involved in the operation of this mechanism and to what degree. In fact, Albert and Obler (1978) were forced to conclude from their analysis of the literature on the subject that "multiple processes are involved in the conscious or unconscious decision to switch from one language to another, either in processing incoming language or in producing language" (p. 214) and that the phenomenon cannot be merely explained in terms of brain functioning. Thus, focusing on the description of the linguistic and psycholinguistic characteristics of the mechanism may provide us with important information of the ways the mechanism is triggered and the factors associated with the activation, as previously discussed (Javier & Marcos, 1989). In this context, we will examine again different factors that are involved in switching at different times and in different degrees. As you will see, code-switching is not a helter-skelter process but it is rather organized and follows very distinct and clearly delineated sets of rules of operation, albeit automatically executed.

Factors Affecting Switching

Two basic sets of factors have been suggested to contribute to the activation or deactivation of the switching mechanism in bilinguals. The first set of factors (structural linguistic factors) refers to conditions inherent in the language itself or "linguistically determined conditions" that tend to facilitate and/or constrain the switching of the languages (Lipski, 1978; Wakefield et al., 1975; Weinreich, 1974). The facilitation and/or restraint of the switching mechanism can also be caused by the second set of factors (nonstructural or extralinguistic factors). These factors refer to the more social and psychological conditions affecting language switching (Greenfield & Fishman, 1975; Javier, 1996; Perez-Foster, 1996; Shaffer, 1978).

Structural Linguistic Factors

In reference to the first set of conditions, Weinreich (1974) observed that code switching tends to occur more frequently in situations around three distinct conditions:

1. When the "designative quality" of the vocabulary corresponding to any of the languages is inadequate to name new things, persons, personal experiences and concepts.
2. When the "low frequency" of certain words in any of the bilingual vocabularies makes it necessary for the speaker to search for replacements in the other language.
3. When the bilingual semantic fields are "insufficiently differentiated."

An example of this third condition is the permanent incorporation of the German word *kranz* (wreath) in the vocabulary of an Italian–German bilingual to differentiate between "crown" and "wreath," for both of which the word "corona" is used (Weinreich, 1974, pp. 56–61). The Arabic words *Jihad*, and *Al Qaeda* now often found in the American lexicon and brought about by the war in Afghanistan, are examples of the first condition (Peraino & Thomas, 2002).

Switching is not likely to occur, however, within what Lipski (1978) refers to as "unbreakable" or "atomic" linguistic structures. He observed that it is a very rare occurrence in verbal expression for a bilingual to split, for example, main verbs from auxiliaries, such as "*yo* must *esperar*" (I must wait); subjects from verbs, such as "*ellos* gave" (they gave); and adjectives from nouns, such as "*su favorito* spot" (his favorite spot). He observed instead that the switching of codes is mainly facilitated between the "constituent boundaries," provided that the syntactical structures of the sentences involved are of nearly perfect congruence, especially in those portions falling after the switching. An example provided by Lipski of a nearly identical syntactical structure can be seen in the sentence,

> +*Me duelen las manos porque las traigos quemadas*/from holding the steering wheel.

The above sentence is made up of the sentence

> +*me duelen las manos porque las traigos tan quemadas/de (por) agarrar el timón (volante),*

and the sentence

> +my hands hurt because they are so scorched/from holding the steering wheel (Lipski, 1978, p. 259).

Lipski claims that the phrases after the slashes are seen as having nearly identical syntactical structures and, therefore, switching is facilitated. This was experimentally demonstrated by Wakefield et al. (1975) with a group of Korean–English and Spanish–English bilinguals. These investigators exposed these two groups of bilinguals to selections concerning various themes, presented visually and auditorily. The subjects were then asked to evaluate, in the mode of the presentation (visual or auditory), the truthfulness or falseness of a series of sentences concerning the content of the stories by pressing a button. These sentences were arranged beginning in the native language of the subjects and then switching to English or vice versa. In addition, the language switch occurred either at the major constituent boundary or within one of the major constituents. These individuals exhibited longer response time when the flow of the sentence was disturbed. That is, "longer response times resulted from the sentences in which the language change occurred within a constituent" (p. 14).

The fact that the proper and faster switching of the languages occurs in those instances where the structural characteristics of the languages involved are respected can be construed as further evidence of the language independence phenomenon. In fact, the structural characteristics of the languages seem to encourage in bilinguals and polyglots the establishment and maintenance of a coordinate relationship between or among their languages. To speak of one unitary linguistic system, the language should be completely and easily translatable and equally switchable at any level of the sentences and not only at the constituent boundaries. In addition, no difference should exist between a subject's response to a unilingual and a bilingual list with various switches. This, however, is not the case with Wakefield et al.'s subjects. In the same vein, Kolers' (1968) study demonstrated that his French–English subjects needed more time to read (aloud) a series of mixed passages than to read (aloud) unilingual ones. Similarly, Macnamara and Kushnir (1971) found that their subjects responded (true or false) fastest to material presented unilingually in their strong language, next fastest to material presented unilingually in the weakest language, next to material containing one switch between languages, and next to material with two switches. The response was slowest to material containing three language switches.

It appears, then, that the switching of the languages runs counter to what Macnamara and Kushnir refer to as "psychological 'inertia' " (1971, p. 486). The fact that the switching of the languages takes time suggests that its occurrence should serve an important function for the individual doing the switching. It is our contention that these switches convey something very specific to the listener above and beyond the purely linguistic communication. Thus, "how" the languages are shifted, "with whom" these shifts are made, "where" these are made, and "at what point" in the conversation a shift occurs may be used by the individual to communicate something about his or her relation to the interlocutor, attitude and feeling about the topic of the conversation, feelings about the locale where the interaction takes place, beliefs, and the like. Shaffer (1978) and Clyne (1967) stated that these factors, which they call "situational appropriateness" or "extralinguistic" factors, tend to have a direct influence on the whole language-switching process.

Relevant to this point is Rubin's (1962) observation in Paraguay that Spanish was reserved for more formal interactions whereas Güaraní, was only used for the most intimate and informal social interactions. For example, young men used Spanish when they first started to court their sweethearts but shifted to Güaraní, when they became more intimate. A similar phenomenon was reported by Blom (1971), who studied the linguistic interactions of Norwegian subjects. These individuals were observed to use the dialect Ranamål for the more informal or intimate interactions (e.g., family, friend), switching into Bokmål for more formal interactions (e.g., jobs, school, and other professional situations). Thus, these authors claimed that as these individuals' definitions of the situations changed (situational switching) and their attitude toward the topic of the conversation changed (metaphorical switching), so did their languages.

Extralinguistic and Affective Factors

It is clear from our previous discussion that language switching cannot be explained solely as a linguistic phenomenon and only when considering the individual's emotional needs are we in a position to have a better understanding of the phenomenon. A case in point is the work by Greenfield and Fishman (1975) who selected 41 hypothetical situations as representatives of the domains of family, friendship, religion, education, and employment. They then asked a group of Spanish–English Puerto Rican subjects to imagine themselves in each of the 41 situations and to assume that they and all other persons mentioned knew Spanish and English equally well. Each of the situations included an *'interlocutor,'* a *'locale'* where the interaction was assumed to take place, and a *'topic'* of discussion. The subjects' task was to indicate their language preference for each of the situations. Again, Rubin's and Blom's findings were corroborated by the results in the present study. These authors found that Spanish was more often selected in intimacy-related situations than in those stressing status. By contrast, English was claimed more often in situations consisting of education- and occupation-related persons, places, and topics than in those that consisted of corresponding components associated with religion. Moreover, Spanish was claimed most frequently in situations consisting of "parents" and least frequently in situations consisting of "teacher" or "employer." Spanish was used with intermediate frequency in those situations consisting of "friend" or "priest."

The above studies clearly suggest that the individual tends to develop different relationships toward his or her languages and that "when," "where," and "with whom" the languages are switched reflects these relationships. As the individual shifts between or among languages, he or she relates to one of the languages, usually the mother tongue, as the bearer of emotional and intimate interactions. The other language, usually the second language, becomes associated with more formal and less intimate interactions (Blom, 1971; Greenfield & Fishman, 1975). Furthermore, if one of the languages carries a greater "social desirability" status, the individual may also shift his or her languages to communicate social preference. Such is the case reported by Fishman (1965) for the language use in Belgium. He observed that French in that country enjoys the most prestigious status while Flemish is considered to have a much lower and less desirable status. Consequently, a Fleming would only use French when in contact with the larger society. Similarly, in the United States, English is the language of social and professional advancement and thus enjoys a certain preference over any other languages when these factors are operative. Spanish is also becoming a language of preference in business and professional situations in some sectors of the United States because of the increased demand of that language as a result of increase in the Latino population and the economic and political power progressively associated with this population in the United States and in Latin America (US Census, 2000).

Greenfield and Fishman's findings that one of the languages is preferred for intimate situations and when deeply emotional contents are to be communicated (as in the case reported by Rubin) found further corroborations in the work of Buxbaum (1949), Stengel (1939), Greenson (1950), Javier (1989, 1996), and Perez-Foster (1996), referred to earlier. Since the individual's early emotions are assumed to originate early in life in interactions parental figures, and since the learning of the language also occurs during this period, it is not surprising that the mother tongue becomes the sole bearer of these emotions and the language that best communicates experiences in which these emotions operate (Javier, 1996). In this regard, psychoanalytic psychotherapy, which has as its tenets the resolution of conflicts through the analysis of the patient's verbalization of materials presumed to be of pregenital nature (first few years of life), is expected to become more affective when the "pregenital tongue," or "the mother tongue," is utilized as the language of treatment. Greenson (1950) observed, in this context, that deeply seated infantile conflicts in his patients could only be fully revealed during treatment when verbalized in the language in association with which such conflicts developed. Buxbaum (1949) states that only when the individual verbalizes such conflicts in the mother tongue, "the language in which they occurred makes them become real; speaking of them in any other language renders them unreal." Thus, speaking in the mother tongue during treatment, "becomes the vehicle of reviving the past and releasing unconscious wishes and emotions into consciousness" (p. 286).

What emerges from the above data is the fact that the emotionality of the content being communicated will trigger switching of the linguistic codes depending upon the subject's intention to communicate or his or her need to avoid experiencing uncomfortable affects.

Role of Stress in Code-Switching

Guided by these observations of code-switching, we wanted to examine more systematically not only the extent and the manner in which stress or strong emotion affects language switching behavior in bilingual individuals but also how this phenomenon is present in monolinguals as well. We believe that linguistic code-switching is a more general phenomenon in language behavior. In the case of monolinguals, code-switching can be seen in the context of one language while for bilinguals we also look at between language switching. In Chapter 2, I attempted to provide a general description of language development, with particular emphasis on bilingual organization. At this point, I want to emphasize the cognitive progression from phonological to semantic organization that characterizes language development. Thus, the first level of organization is around the sound of the word, while semantic organization represents a higher and more sophisticated level of linguistic organization. When an individual's natural language behavior is disrupted as a result of a high emotion, stress, or other conditions, the concept of code-switching also applies intralinguistically. Thus, when the individual becomes temporarily unable to process language at the semantic level and becomes more interested in the phonemic quality of the linguistic production, such a switching will certainly impact on the ability to process and categorize information around him or her at a higher and more abstract cognitive level. If this were to happen, it can only occur under conditions that disrupt the natural functional environment in the organism that also result in a disruption in the cognitive process.

A number of investigators attempted to create experimentally such a condition to then examine how language function is affected. Among these investigators we find the work of Razran (1939), Riess (1940), Bridger (1970) with monolingual subjects and of Javier and Alpert (1986) and Javier and Marcos (1989), with bilingual subjects. In 1939 Razran, for instance, published a study in which he sought to investigate linguistic (semantic) generalization through the utilization of the classical conditioning technique. In the first part of his experiment, he conditioned six subjects to a series of words (e.g., style, urn, freeze, and surf) and flashed short sentences on a screen while the subjects were eating. Conditioned salivation developed to these words and sentences. For the purpose of testing generalization, different words semantically and phonemically related to the conditioned lists of words (e.g., fashion, stile, earn, vase, frieze, chill, serf, and wave) and different sets of sentences were used in the second session. His findings for the single words indicate greater generalization for semantically related words than for phonemically related words.

Notwithstanding the serious methodological flaws found in Razran' study, his findings were later replicated by Riess (1940), who utilized the same set of words used by Razran but introduced the galvanic skin response (GSR) to measure generalization. In addition, he also used a loud buzzer as an unconditioned stimulus. The buzzer is not only of a different nature (auditory vs. visual) but is clearly a more aversive or noxious condition than the one used by Razran. In the first experimental session, each subject was exposed to 50 stimulus words, presented seriatim. Four of these words were conditioned at a second experimental session to the sound of a buzzer. The list was constructed to include words semantically and phonemically related to the four major stimulus words, and the GSRs for each word were recorded. In the second experimental session, the stimulus word was presented in association with the buzzer in an attempt to condition the word to the sound of the buzzer. The criterion used by this author to determine if conditioning had taken place was that the stimulus word alone had to produce a GSR of at least three times the amplitude of the reaction prior to the conditioning on three out of four successive trials. Immediately following the attainment of the criterion, the homophone and the synonym for each conditioned word were presented five times, each in a random order. His findings indicate that the carryover to the semantically related words was consistently greater than to the phonemically related words. Since this study still suffers from the kinds of methodological problems that ail Razran's study, the findings have to be viewed with caution (Javier & Marcos, 1989).

Contrary to Razran's and Riess's findings, Luria and Vinogradova (1959) showed that the introduction of experimental conditions such as hypnosis, or the administration of chloral hydrate, or fatigue produced a shift in the nature of generalization in the subjects from semantically to phonemically related words. Unfortunately, because of the lack of information as to the ways in which these studies were carried out, it is not possible to evaluate them properly. Nonetheless, one can at least conclude that these conditions were of such a kind (abnormal) as to have produced a qualitative change in the linguistic responses of these subjects from semantically to phonemically related words.

Bridger (1970), Vygostky (1962), and Luria and Yudovich (1968) claim that one's responses to the phonemic aspects of the language are of a different kind and at a more primitive level than responses to the semantic aspect of the language. As discussed earlier, the semantic aspect of language is considered to be associated with and to mediate the more symbolic and abstract aspects of the mental process, while the phonemic aspect is considered to be associated with and to mediate the more concrete aspect of cognition. It appears, then, that the conditions studied by Luria and Vinogradova also produced a definite shift (primitivization) in the cognitive functioning of their subjects.

Bridger (1970) subsequently demonstrated that stressful anxiety-provoking conditions also produce the same linguistic shift in generalization found by Luria and Vinogradova. Bridger operationally defined stress as the change in the GSR that followed a signal of forthcoming painful (electrical shock) stimulations. Unlike Razran's and Riess's studies, however, Bridger's experimental design included controls that allow for a clearer interpretation of his findings. For instance, his list of words was presented orally and included words semantically and phonemically unrelated to the conditioned stimulus so that the effect of generalization is less equivocally observed. In addition, to determine the extent to which stress affects generalization, he included two different intensities of electric shocks and compared the effect in the generalization of the conditioned response.

For his study, Bridger divided his subjects into three groups (A, B, and C) of 20 subjects each. The stimulus words were "boat," "door," "ship," "cloud," and "skip" and were presented to the subjects orally. "Ship" was the conditioned stimulus while "skip" is a word phonemically related to "ship" and "boat" is a word semantically related to "ship." "Door" is a neutral word unrelated to "ship."

Bridger's findings indicate, among other things, that stress or strong emotional affect (strong electric shock) produces a relative increase in phonemic as compared to semantic generalization, thus confirming the findings of Luria and Vinogradova. That is, this intense stimulus forced a violation of the normal linguistic processing, thus encouraging a more primitive (phonemic) linguistic response. The lesser the electric shock the more the generalization to the semantically related words. In addition, semantic generalization only occurred in those subjects who expected shock reinforcement with the conditioned word "boat" because of its relation with the word "ship." He concluded that the generalization to the phonemically related words occurs unconsciously and under conditions of stress, whereas generalization to semantically related words takes place more consciously and under more normal conditions.

Bridger's findings were also replicated with bilinguals by Javier and Alpert (1986) and by Javier and Marcos (1989) using the same paradigm to study linguistic generalization across the bilingual languages. We were concerned with studying the extent to which, and the manner in which, stress affects across language generalization. We were also concerned with the extent to which the language independence phenomenon (or the assumed functional separation of the languages) may inhibit generalization of the effect of stress across languages. For this purpose, a group of Spanish–English coordinate bilinguals were subjected to conditions similar to the ones undergone by Bridger's groups. As described by Bridger (1970), these conditions allow for the investigation of stress under an unconscious condition, as the subject is not provided with any information about the stimulus contingencies and reinforcement expectations. For each group, one of two different stimulus words [one in each language: "bote" (boat) and "house"] was paired with one of two different intensities of a buzzer sound (stressful condition). The GSR provided a measure of the effect of the conditioning (assumed to be stressful) and later of the extent of generalization. To study generalization, two bilingual lists with words semantically and phonemically related in both languages ("barco," "dote," "ship," "butter," "mesa," and "candy" for the first list, or "casa," "home," "mouse," "jaulas," "toro," and "apple" for the second list) to the conditioned stimuli were included, as well as words from both languages unrelated to the stimulus words (CS: "bote" for the first list and "house" for the second list).

We found a differential impact of the buzzer on the functional separation of the language. Although linguistic generalization was present in both languages and buzzer conditions, the mild buzzer condition encouraged more generalization in the language opposite to the language of the stimulus. The more intense stressful condition tended to encourage more generalization in the language of the stimulus and hence preserving the functional separation of the languages, as discussed earlier. This suggests that under conditions of mild stress, where there is less disorganization of the cognitive process, code-switching is more likely.

Effect of Stress on Learning

The implications of these findings for learning are enormous, suggesting that the transfer of information across language is more likely to occur when the level of stress/anxiety is within manageable range. When a child is in a classroom situation where it also has to deal with too stressful emotions, learning is expected to be affected in that not only the linguistic organization of the material is affected, but the cross-language transferability of the information learned as well. We have observed the impact of conditions of stress in cognitive development and academic performance in children suffering from different levels of lead intoxication, a condition that tends to produce physiological stress, neurological complication, and general discomfort in the children (Needleman, Schell, Bellinger, Leviton & Allred, 1990). The higher the lead levels the more likely that serious language function will be affected (CDC, 1991), including the ability to learn in a second language. In later chapters, we will be discussing this issue further.

Similarly, a home and community environment where a great deal of tension is present and where the child's personal and emotional survival may be at risk is less likely to be conducive to learning and to the transfer of information cross-linguistically. Thus, children suffering from severe poverty, unstable home environments, divorce, community violence, child abuse, etc. are more likely to exhibit learning problems, including language-specific difficulties (Javier & Camacho-Gingerich, 2004). We can extend this analysis to include children living in war-torn communities (e.g., Lebanon, Iraq, in Sudan) without a stable family and sociopolitical environment due to instability of the major institutions responsible for the care of these children. The resulting loss of parental and family support (due to illness or death) is likely to make their environment toxic for learning.

Conclusion

It is clear that language switching is governed by specific linguistic mechanisms and structures that determine the extent and nature of language switching likely to occur. It is also clear that language switching is used to communicate specific information about the speaker to the listener; this process is partly determined by the nature of emotional material and cognition involved. Stress and anxiety-provoking situations may trigger language switching, leading to the development of language-specific memories and to conditions that could make the level of accessibility of these memories/information problematic in the future. Whether these language-specific memories are accessible in the other language is a function of how these memories were organized in the specific-language, the nature of the language-specific memories, the specific language systems involved in these memories, the kinds and extent of bilingual organization characterizing the individual's linguistic organization, and the level of linguistic proficiency in each language of the bilingual individual.

The issue to consider here with regard to learning in general, and learning in a second language in particular, is that a situation of too much stress or tension is likely to affect learning and the development of learning strategies that can facilitate transference of information across languages. When the conditions are too stressful and traumatic, there can be a partial or complete shutdown of the normal learning process and thus making some language-specific memories temporally, or more or less permanently, inaccessible in another language. This issue of linguistically-influenced memory inaccessibility is discussed more fully in the next chapter.

5
Bilingual Memory and the Language of Affect

Studies of memory accessibility have a long tradition in the behavioral sciences because of the importance of memory in most aspects of the individual's cognitive development (Baddeley, 1991). Memory allows the individual to remember and organize events and experiences of various kinds that accumulate through his or her life cycle. It allows the individual to organize and categorize information received from different (internal and external) sources. The importance of assessing the nature of memory organization that is possible in bilingualism is further highlighted by the fact that there are different kinds of memories possible (such as memory for places, for objects, events, people, etc.) (Baddeley, 1991; Cohen, 1991; Riccio, Rabinowitz, & Axerold, 1994); that different parts of the brain are involved in these memories (Locke, 1994; Luria, 1973, 1981); and that bilingual languages are intimately involved in the organization and categorization of these memories.

In previous chapters, we have been making references to the many ways the brain is intimately involved in the bilingual languages and cognitive development. At this point, we will focus our attention more carefully on the specific ways as to how the bilingual cognitive development is intimately connected to normal brain function, and, more particularly, on how we develop memories of experiences in the context of the bilingual process. Thus, we will focus in the next section on the neurological aspects of memory, on how we remember in general and how memories are formed in the normal course of human cognitive development. We will then discuss the specific issues related to memory formation in a bilingual context.

Neurological Aspects of Memory

We have been provided with the most awesome structure – the brain – that is involved in all aspects of our lives (Figure 5.1). Every aspect of this structure actively contributes to the development of the most fundamental mental qualities that distinguish humans from nonhumans and that allows us to perceive, to organize experiences, to think, to dream, to feel, to create, and, yes, to remember. The brain has a number of simple and complex mechanisms that allow us to remember every aspect of our experiences that are important (e.g., things that we touch, smell, hear, see, think); simple and complex information are all

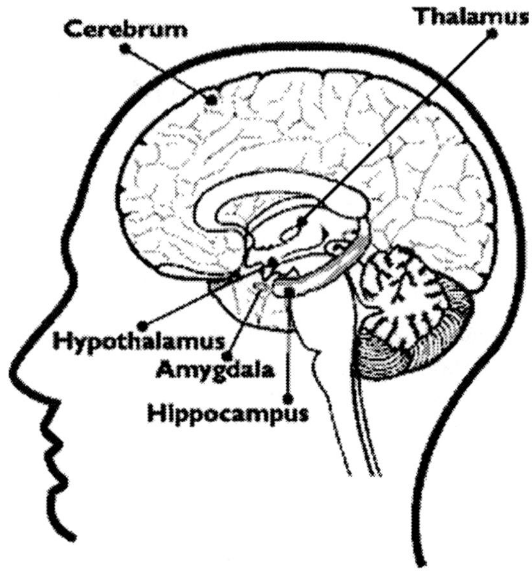

This drawing of a brain cut in half demonstrates some of the brain's internal structures. The amygdala and hippocampus are actually located deep within the brain, but are shown as an overlay in the approximate areas that they are located.

Published by National Institute on Drug Abuse, Mind Over Master Teaching Guide, retrieved from http : //teens.drugabuse.gov/mom/tg_nerves.asp on 11/24/2006.

FIGURE 5.1. Picture of the brain and its structures.
Source:
The **hippocampus** is the part of the limbic system associated with conscious factual/rational (declarative) memories. The hippocampus can store information for either short periods of time or long periods of time depending on the type of information being stored.
The **amygdala** is the part of the limbic system associated with unconscious behavioral/emotional (procedural) memories.
The **thalamus** is part of the limbic system associated with transmission of sensory information to the cerebral cortex.
The **basal ganglia** is a control system for movement and cognitive functions.
The **hypothalamus** is part of the limbic system associated with regulation of body temperature, metabolism and influences certain emotions.
(Luria, 1973)

organized into different storages of information that we can then retrieve as later points as the situations call for.

As defined by Braddeley in his book *Human Memory* (1991),

> Human memory is a system for storing and retrieving information... acquired through our senses. (p. 13)

He went on to say that human memory is not a single unitary system but multiple systems that, working in concert, give a total unity, each with the capacity to store information. Memories are records of percepts that depend on sensory modality. In fact, there is a memory storage associated with each sense. And what is interesting is that,

> The systems range in storage duration from fractions of a second up to a lifetime, and in storage capacity from tiny buffer stores to the long-term memory system that appears to far exceed in capacity and flexibility the largest available computer. (p. 4)

If I were to ask you, the reader, to close your eyes and try to remember the color of a room you just visited and the kinds of chairs in the room, the texture and color of the rugs, etc., your ability to remember these details will be a function of how important it is for you to retrieve these details from the sensory-perceptual storage where they were deposited once perceived. Or if I were to ask someone living in the tropical region to tell me as many kinds of snow as he/she can remember, this list will be much smaller than the one an Eskimo will give, who is forced, by necessity (survival needs), to be very familiar with different kinds of snow. Different kinds of snow may require different response schemata from individuals living in a snow-bound environment so as to ensure their survivability. If these individuals miss the signs for snowstorms or ice-storms, are unable to identify from where and when to retrieve their food, what snow is best to walk on and which one should be avoided, how to keep warm etc. are likely to have a difficult time surviving in that environment. Similarly, someone coming to a new city may become more hyper-attentive to information about nearby hospitals than any other information, if suffering from a recurrent medical condition that is likely to require medical attention. In the same context, individuals with a specialty (e.g., computer programmer, car mechanic, pulmonary specialist, English teacher, physicist, speech and language pathologist, brain surgeon) will require to have access to their specialty-specific information in their memory storage in order to function successful in their professions.

But how do we develop our memories? Normally, information from various sources comes the brain to be processed (such as when an individual hears the sound of an oncoming car, finally sees a car coming at a relative fast speed as he/she is crossing the street). This information is then processed following a specific and preditermined path. This information is organized as new information or belonging to a category of information already in memory. Part of this organization also involves the processing of the information in terms of the degree of urgency requiring immediate response (like the example of the individual attempting to cross the street referred to above; this individual has to decide if the car is going too fast and is likely to hit him/her or if the driver is showing any sign that s/he has seen the pedestrian and has enough time to stop the vehicle on time); or requiring less immediate response (i. e., the pedestrian is not within the range of being hit by the car and hence not at risk). The capacity of the brain to assess the nature of these types of information is one of its most important abilities for our survival. If what is requires from the brain is too involved and intense, and more complex than what the individual is accustomed to (such as, following the example of the car, when several cars are coming at once at high speed and the individual does not see a clear way out), the individual may find it difficult to respond and could shut down (i. e., become immobilized). That is, it goes into a protective mode, or a desperate attempt to protect itself from being too overwhelmed. The information may remain partly unprocessed and the memory of the event encapsulated in a separate storage, at the sensory motor level.

Harry Stack Sullivan (1953), as discussed in Chapter 2, provides us with the most vivid example of the way the mind works in a situation that is too intense and painful (e.g., a traumatic event) for the system to integrate as part of previously gathered memories. He was referring to the emotional development, but in the final analysis, he was mainly referring to the work of the brain as it relates to bio-physiological and emotional demands. According to this author, experiences are organized and remembered along two basic dimensions: Those where the individual's basic physiological and emotional needs create an increase in physiological and emotional tension in the organism (i.e., loss of the natural biochemical equilibrium – as when one is hungry – and/or when anxiety sets in, in the psychological realm) that is quickly reduced by the response of the external environment (i.e., when the mother covers the body of the child that is too cold or gives milk to the child that is hungry). These types of experiences are organized as "good-me" experiences or experiences of well-being and become part of the self-definition and the way the world is perceived (as affirming/supportive/benign). When the response to these needs is not forthcoming for any number of reasons (as it happens in an environment where the mother or mothering one may be emotionally and/or physically unavailable – like in the case of a mother with substance abuse, poor mental health, or in situations when the child is placed in an orphanage.) tension will set in. This tension is experienced psychologically as anxiety and the individual is then forced to organize these experiences in the memory system as part of the "bad me" experience, or experience to be avoided. The organism's need to protect itself against tension/anxiety will force a clear distinction between these two types of memories. When the experience is too intense and personally too threatening to be organized along these two dimensions (such as in the case of a traumatic event, experience of child abuse, physical abuse, domestic violence, terrorist attacks), the individual will tend to organize these experiences along the "not-me" experience, dissociated from the rest of the memory system, inaccessible to consciousness. So, one may hear an individual exposed to a traumatic event not being able to remember many aspects of these types of events.

But let's take a look at the picture of the brain (Fig. 5.1) to see how these and other experiences are formed.

The great Russian scholar Alexander Romanovich Luria (1973) describes three principal functional units of the brain in his book *The Working Brain*, which was later supported by a number of neurological findings (Dubois, et al. 1995; Petrides, 1995)

1. Unit for regulating tone or waking and mental states
2. Unit for obtaining, processing, and storing information arriving from the outside world
3. Unit for programming, regulating, and verifying mental activity.

These units participate in any type of mental activity and they follow a very specific hierarchical structure. They consist of at least three different cortical zones built one above the other (Figure 5.2):

1. The primary (projection) area that receives impulses or sends impulses from the periphery (subcortex and brain stem – reticular formation).
2. Secondary (projection association) area where incoming information is processed or programs are prepared [midbrain, located in the lateral regions of the neocortex on the convex surface of the hemispheres, of which it occupies the posterior regions, including the visual (occipital), auditory (temporal), and general sensory (parietal) regions].
3. Tertiary (zones of overlapping) area where the latest system of the cerebral hemispheres develop and are responsible in humans for the most complex

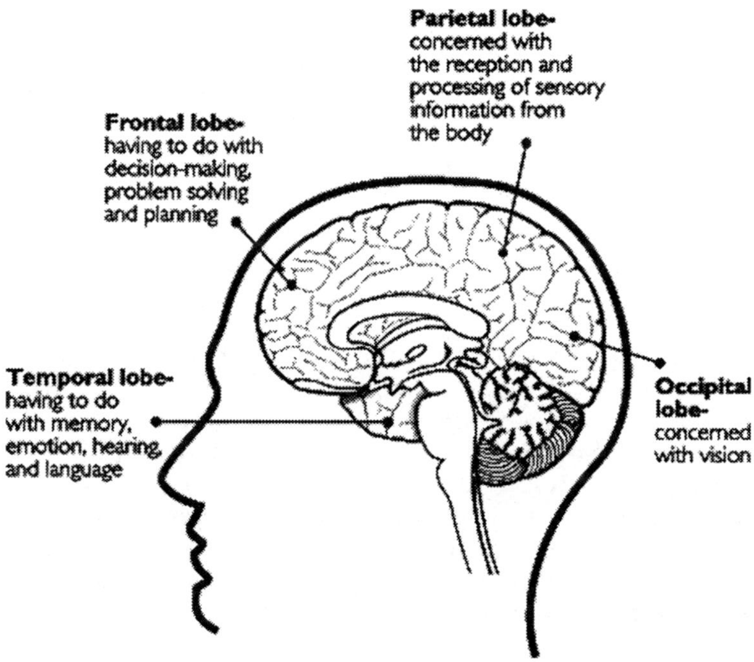

Published by National Institute on Drug Abuse, Mind Over Matter Teaching Guide, retrieved from http : //teens.drugabuse.gov/mom/tg_nerves.asp on 11/24/2006.

FIGURE 5.2. A cross-section of the brain and its structures.

forms of mental activities, requiring the concentrated participation of many cortical areas (located in the frontal lobes, or more precisely the prefrontal divisions of the brain).

The beauty of this is that these units working in concert allow for multiple and progressively more complex memories to develop. Thus, the process of memory development can be sketchily described as follows:

- From simple sensory memory (formed from what we see, hear, touch, taste, smell, and moving through the visual, auditory, tactile, gustatory, olfactory, kinesthetic cortical structures), information is organized and compared with other information that had been previously received from the environment. New information that cannot be organized within previously organized information (memories) is organized in a separate structure.
- Associative links are developed among all the information gathered that get progressively more complex, ending in the creation of thoughts and creativity of various kinds.
- At the highest level of mental process, language is involved in the organization and categorization of the experience that is stored in memory.

A lesion in any of these cortical areas produces different kinds of memory disturbances, depending on if it is in the limbic system (nonspecific memory loss), the midbrain, or the more developed part of the brain responsible for more sophisticated and complex processes (loss of intention and planning). Let's take a closer look at each of these areas individually to see how these areas contribute to the whole memory organization. Again, Luria (1973) provides us with the most eloquent and clear description of these different brain systems.

Unit for Regulating Tone and Waking and Mental States

All organized and goal-directed activity requires that the brain has optimal level of alertness or cortical tone or optimal neuro-dynamics. Like if you are at a conference or listening to someone present information at a time that you feel particularly sleepy, some of the information being communicated may be lost because it may never get to be fully received and processed by the brain. But if person presenting were to raise his or her voice or screamed, you will immediately open your eyes and investigate what may have occurred and if you judged it to be of personal irrelevance, you may go back to a sleepy mode; if you found it to be a dangerous situation, it will demand immediate action and the cerebral cortex will be at the optimal level of responsiveness. This is part of the survival mechanism of the organism.

This capacity of the brain to respond to novel stimuli in this manner is what Luria (1973) refers to as the "law of strength." According to Luria (1973), the cortex is guided by the law of strength where a response to external stimuli can occur only if a state of optimal excitation is maintained, where every strong (or biologically significant) stimulus evokes a strong response, while every weak stimulus evokes a weak response. According to Luria (1973), during this period there is a concentration of nervous processes, there is a balance between excitation and inhibition, and there is a high mobility of the nervous processes so that it is easy to change from one activity to another.

In a state of lowered cortical tone (during sleep), the normal relationship between excitation and inhibition is broken, the law of strength is disturbed, and the mobility of the nervous system is lost. Sleep is important for the organism and hence the brain will find ways to create the optimal environment (lowering of the cortical tone) to make it possible for the individual to fall asleep. However, if the external conditions are experienced by the individual as too threatening (e.g., a break-in in the house while one is sleeping, a fire inside the house or an explosion in the proximity of the dwelling), sleep may be disturbed. We normally find these conditions when the individual may have experienced a traumatic event that was physically and/or emotionally threatening.

The brain system responsible for that activity is the brain stem, particularly the reticular formation (Figures 5.2 and 5.3) whose function is to send the information to the rest of the cortex, demanding action. It influences the rest of the cortex but is also influenced and regulated by the cortex. What the reticular formation does is to gradually change the tone level of the cortex little by little, thus modulating the whole state of the nervous system. In a state of sleep the system basically slows down all systems (almost like dimming the light to cut down all stimuli so that the brain does not feel compelled to respond). That is, it reduces the level of excitation that is sent to the cortex. It also inhibits the information that may come from the higher cortex so that the reticular formation becomes central to the whole memory operation by changing the tone of the cortex (ascending reticular formation) and thus making it possible for memory to be developed and stored at that level. But under the influence of the cortex, it is regulated and modified by changes taking place in the cortex (descending reticular formation). In this manner it adapts itself readily to the environmental conditions and the required course of activity.

Damage to this section of the brain is non-specific because it affects the whole system and memory of information coming from the environment through the senses modes. As described by Luria (1973), it could have also an impact on specific activities, such as certain orienting reflexes (which is so important in investigative activity) and inborn behavioral systems or systems of instinctive (or unconditioned reflex) food getting and sexual behavior. Orienting reflex allows for comparison between novel situations and old ones to determine if a response is necessary. Habituation takes place when the individual is exposed repeatedly to the same stimulus and thus looses its novelty. Under this condition, it sends the information to the rest of the organism that special mobilization of the different systems is no longer necessary. According to Luria (1973), a patient with a lesion in the limbic system may appear fatigued and depressed, bordering on indifference, and the ability to provide a lucid account of his or her history is affected and so is his or her orientation.

We are reminded, in this context, of a patient who was the victim of a severe fire at her house resulting in serious burns in her hands and legs that required a long hospitalization. She lost consciousness and was in a coma for about a month. Even months later, she was rather confused about what had happened and how she was able to get out of her building. On returning to the apartment, she was very afraid of staying in that apartment and became extremely sensitive to smell and found herself smelling smoke even if it was from a car engine across the street. This can be considered a necessary and natural behavior from a woman who was greatly affected by her not noticing early enough that the building was on fire and full of smoke. Since there is no known damage to her brain, this reaction is expected to disappear as habituation sets in.

Unit for Receiving, Analyzing and Storing Information

As indicated earlier, this unit is located in close proximity to the superior cortex (see Figures 5.1–5.3). It is the second brain system and is located in the lateral regions of the neocortex or the convex surface of the hemispheres, of which it occupies the posterior regions, including the visual (occipital), auditory (temporal), and general sensory (parietal) regions (Luria, 1973). This functional unit of brain has high modal specificity. That is, that its component parts are highly specialized (neurons of afferent layer IV) for the reception of visual,

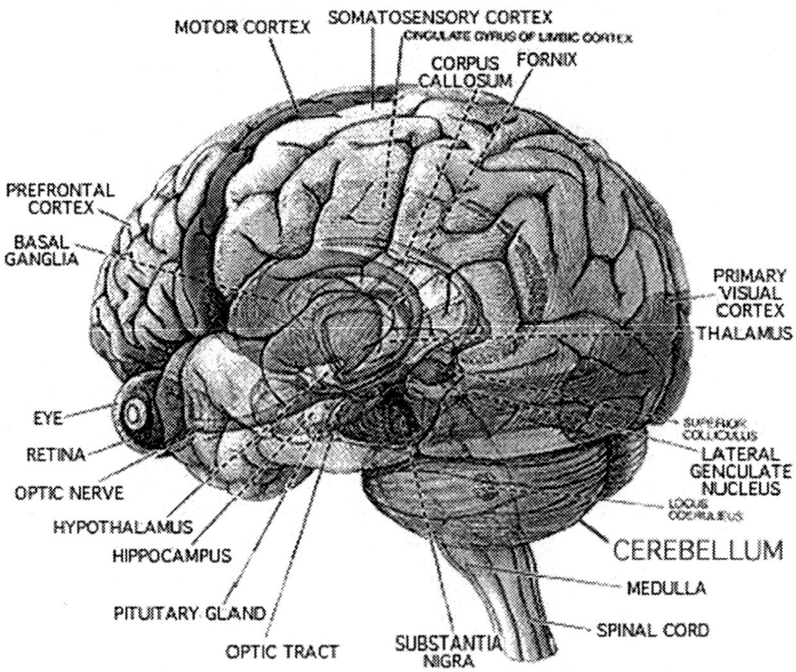

FIGURE 5.3. Picture of principal structures of the brain involved in memory formation.

auditory, vestibular, or general sensory information. It is also the central system of gustatory and olfactory reception. That is, it also consists of cells of the associative layers II and III of the cortex.

The more refined part of this region (its tertiary zone that is located in the superior and inferior zones of the parietal region) is involved in the conversion of concrete perception into abstract thinking, which proceeds in the form of internal schemes and for the memorizing of the organized experience. That is, it is not only for the reception and coding of information but for its storage.

In order to accomplish this function this second brain unit is guided by three basic laws:

1. Law of hierarchical structure of the cortical zones; or primary, secondary, tertiary cortical zones dealing progressively with more complex information.
2. Law of diminishing specificity of the hierarchically arranged cortical zones, composing from more modal specificity to less (from neurons of layer IV to layers III and II).
3. Law of progressive lateralization of functions in both hemispheres.

Regarding the third law, for instance, we can see how the left hemisphere (in right-handers) begins to play an essential role not only in the cerebral organization of speech but also in the cerebral organization of all higher forms of cognitive activity, connected with speech (i.e., perception organized into logical schemes, active verbal memory, and logical thought).

Unit for Programming Regulation and Verification of Activity

The brain structure for this functional unit is located in the anterior regions of the hemispheres, anterior to the precentral gyrus (see Figures 5.1–5.3). According to Luria (1973), the outlet for this unit is the motor cortex with layer V neurons that contains the giant pyramidal cells, fibers from which run to the spinal motor nuclei, and from there to the muscles, forming the parts of the great pyramidal track. That is, it has a very rich system of connections both with lower levels of the brain (i.e., the medial and ventral nuclei, pulvinar of the thalamus,) and with virtually all other parts of the cortex. The most important part of this third functional unit is the frontal lobes, or precisely, the prefrontal divisions of the brain.

This part of the brain (prefrontal regions) does not mature until very late in ontogeny and not until the child has reached the age of 4–7 years do they become prepared for actions. In fact, research shows a sharp increase by age 3 1/2–4 and again when 7–8 years old it experiences another jump (Dubois et al., 1995; Luria, 1973).

The connections are two-way and are particularly favorable for the reception and synthesis of the complex system of afferent impulses arriving from all parts of the brain and for the organization of efferent impulses so that they can regulate these structures.

This unit is responsible for the organization of conscious activity. According to Luria (1973), it is the site where the human mind acquires the most refined power and where intentions are created, plans are formed, actions are programmed, their performance inspected, behaviors regulated so that they conform to the original plan and programs. Finally, the individual verifies his or her conscious activity, comparing the effects of his or her actions with the original intentions and corrects any mistake, if appropriate.

According to Luria (1973), this is in fact a superstructure above all other parts of the cerebral cortex so that they perform a far more universal function of general regulation of behavior than that performed by the posterior associative center of the second functional unit. For humans, the regulation of functions takes place with the close participation of speech. Damage to this part disturbs the whole human activity having to do with intentions and plans, as well as regulation of mental activity and verification of its course and results. Memory for these activities is affected, giving a sense of no clear purpose for his or her action and mental activity.

For additional discussion of these issues, the reader is also encouraged to review two important publications on the subject. One edited by Grafman, Holyoak, and Boller (1995) entitled *Structure and Functions of the Human Prefrontal Cortex* and the second edited by Tallal, Galaburda, Llinas, and Euler (1993) entitled *Temporal Information Processing in the Nervous System.*

Since language is the single most important development that allows for the most comprehensive and refined organization of memory of human experience, we will now turn our discussion to how important memories are organized linguistically. We will then take a look at the kinds of challenges individuals who possess more than one language to organize their various experiences and develop memories bring to the discussion on the subject.

Developmental Factors in Memory Formation

There are specific developmental factors that have a direct impact on the extent to which an event can be remembered. These include neurological and linguistic factors referred to earlier. For instance, researchers have identified several reasons why very young children cannot remember an earlier experience:

1. They lack the neurological maturity to encode adequately their experiences.
2. They lack the linguistic ability to encode their experiences verbally.
3. They lack the schemas within which they can represent and organize event memories (Cohen, 1989; Schachtel, 1947).
4. They may have been using encoding strategies that do not help them to elaborate and enrich the memory representation with semantic association.
5. They may be encoding memories in ways that are inappropriate for the retrieval processes used at a later age, and thus it becomes a matter of inappropriate encoding strategies rather than memory loss (Cohen, 1989; Winograd & Killinger, 1983).

I am reminded of a child who, when an infant, was taken to the house of a friend where he had a slight fall; he cried briefly and was given an ice cream (his favorate treat) to calm him down. He responded quickly to the ice cream and proceeded to refer to the experience as great. A few years later, when the parents were making reference to the experience, the child had no recollection of the experience or of having gone to the specific location where the experience took place, although he continues to have a wonderful relationship with the family's friend. This is not an unusual occurrence, as children and even adults are likely to remember, forget, or just have a distorted version of an event, although it does not appear to be a specific reason for the memory not to be available. As indicated earlier, it is clear that, under normal circumstances, we only remember information that is important for the organism/individual to survive organically, cognitively, and psychologically (Baddeley, 1991; Luria, 1973). This is the reason why information becomes organized into categories that can later be recalled when the occasion calls for it. The child then remembers that meals are served around a specific time, that getting too close to the stove will result in burns, or not completing his or her homework could result in a bad grade. Later on, one will also be more likely to remember that failing to come on time to work may result in a dismissal when witnessing that others are dismissed for such an infraction. As said earlier, information such as the color of the walls, the fabric of the chair, the number of nails used to secure the walls may be less likely to be remembered if these memories do not have the same level of importance for the individual. Indeed, being concerned with unimportant aspects of the experience and being unable to screen out irrelevant stimuli are considered one of the characteristics of psychological/psychiatric disturbance, including attention deficit disorder and schizophrenia.

Memory of Traumatic Event in Children: Can Memory be Falsified?

Research evidence supporting the view that child memory could be subject to distortion by external influences (see experimental eyewitness studies by Loftus, 1979) has been used to question the extent to which childhood memories of traumatic events, such as sexual and physical abuse, could also be affected in the same manner. But, according to Riccio, Rabinowitz, and Axerold (1994), only when the stimulus attributes, which provide specificity to a memory of an event, are forgotten is it possible for a memory to become malleable, and hence subject to distortion. Thus, when the child is able to remember "wha*t*" the experience was all about, "where" it took place, "who" was involved in the experience, and *"when"* it occurred, the possibility for distortion and forgetting is minimal (Wagenaar, 1986). Forgetting of stimulus attributes, or specific defining characteristics of the experience under consideration, tends to increase with time and hence distortion and false memory then become more possible (Cohen, 1989). Similarly, it appears that a child's temperament could impact on the malleability of memory; inhibited children were found to be more susceptible to suggestion when asked about a past event than were uninhibited children (Schacter, Kagan, & Leichtman, 1995).

What about the case of bilingual individuals which have a dual linguistic organization of their experiences? What kind of memory organization is possible under this condition and what are the factors affecting accessibility of memory in the two languages? If a bilingual is unable to communicate an experience that occurred in the context of one of the languages in his/her other language, does this constitute inaccessibility of the memory? What if the memory can be accessed in one of the languages but the affective component of the experience remains connected to the other language? We propose that, since the memory of an event is composed of the specific memories and cognitions of the event as well as the affective responses to these events, whenever any aspect of the experience is absent, the accessibility to the experience should be considered incomplete. What we are referring to here is the complexity brought about by the unique characteristics of the bilingual phenomenon, discussed earlier with regard to memory organization and the assessment of memory.

Memory Organization in the Bilingual Context

But how are memories organized linguistically when more than one linguistic code is used to categorize and organize the experience? In an attempt to answer this question, three basic memory models have been suggested by various authors who have attempted to decipher structural characteristics of the bilingual memory (Hines, 1978; Kolers, 1963; Lopez & Young, 1974; Thorson, 1980; Tulving & Calotta, 1970):

1. The independent model
2. The interdependent model
3. The interdependent–dependent model

The interdependent model suggests that an individual's experiences and perceptions are organized along unitary linguistic dimensions that are dependent on one another and are relatively accessible in both languages. When experiences and perceptions are organized along separate linguistic dimensions in more than one language, an independent model is assumed to be operational. The interdependent–dependent model refers to a combination of both models (Javier & Marcos, 1989; Kirsner, Smith, Lockhart, King, & Jain, 1984; Smith, 1991). In this regard, Hines (1978) postulated a unitary, common memory structure shared by both languages, with semantic representations remaining interdependent but orthographic and phonemic representations remaining independent.

An example of the types of studies supporting bilingual memory is the one by Kolers' (1963) word association study, which sought to study bilingual memory organization. He investigated the extent to which experiences are either stored in some kind of supralinguistic form common to each of the bilingual's languages or are stored separately and remain specific to the language in which they occur. Three groups of bilingual subjects (native German, Spanish, and Thai) were asked to give associations to a group of English words and words from their respective native languages. Kolers found that words referring to concrete, manipulatable objects (e.g., pencil, chair, finger) tended to elicit similar associations in both languages more often than words referring to abstract states (e.g., freedom, justice, civilization, honor) or emotions (e.g., pain, love, hate, guilt). Words referring to emotional states elicited very dissimilar associations in both languages. He concluded from these data that "experiences and memories of various kinds are not stored in common in some supra-linguistic form but are tagged and stored separately in the language the subject used to define the experience to himself" (p. 300) or herself.

For Paradis (1978), however, it is possible to have one memory storage corresponding to the bilingual's experiential and conceptual information. This memory storage contains mental representations of things and events, properties, and functions of objects, that is, what is known about the world. According to Paradis, the bilingual also has a language store for each of the two languages, each of which is differentially connected to a conceptual store. In the language store, the bilinguals' conceptual features are grouped into units of meaning, which can be said as words or expressions (Grosjean, 1982). Paradis speaks about units of meanings in each of the languages that group together conceptual features in different ways (Figure 5.4).

Thus, according to this conceptualization, a bilingual individual has one conceptual store that is differentially organized depending on which language is used to verbalize an idea, feelings, or experience. Grosjean (1982) suggests that Paradis' conceptualization explains why some words and experiences are

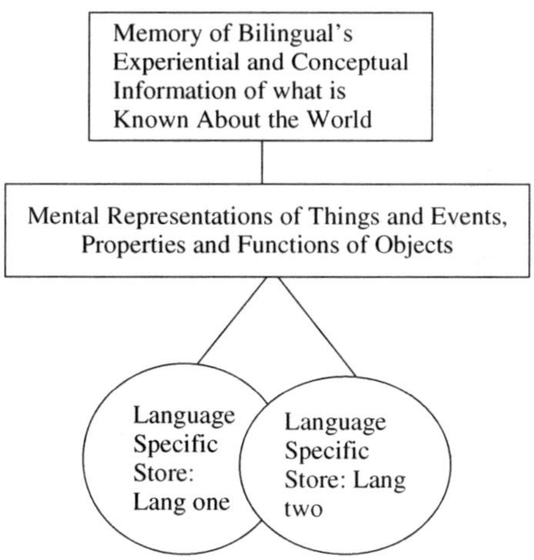

FIGURE 5.4. Memory storage in bilinguals.

difficult to translate into another language because they probably share few conceptual features, whereas other words and their translation equivalents share many conceptual features and hence are easier to translate from one language to another.

The explanatory power of Paradis' memory retrieval model found additional support in De Groot's conceptual feature model (1992a,b, 1993), recently discussed by Schrauf (2000). According to this model, the two languages differentially activate conceptual features. Concrete words correspond to meanings shared across languages and hence are likely to activate the same referents at the conceptual level. The more abstract words, on the other hand, require more contextualization and hence are likely to activate more language-specific features.

The implication for learning is certainly enormous with regard to the generalization of information across languages. It suggests that some information learned in a specific language context is likely to remain language-specific and the other is likely to encourage cross-language generalization. Information learned earlier in life in conjunction with one of the languages is likely to become more or less accessible in both languages only to the extent to which the linguistic concepts utilized to organize and communicate the experience share similar conceptual features in both languages. In general, it is also more likely that certain information is more transferable from one language to the other under conditions of linguistic proficiency regardless of the language-learning environment. This is true for semantic and more concrete information. Emotional and abstract information is likely to be more accessible in connection to the language more closely associated with the development of this specific emotional and abstract information.

Bilingual Memory for Meaningful Information

Language develops and acquires its meaning in relation to important people in our lives and in the context of historical, political, socioeconomic, and ecological conditions that characterize the lives of those upon whom we depend emotionally. Our relationship with the environment, the smell of the land, our mother's caresses, her responses to our calls for food or warmth, the harsh or sweet and embracing voices of our grandparents, the tastes of foods and the succulent juices of fruits, the smells and beauty of the beaches, the hot and dry summer, the rhythmic sound of music, and the different emotions associated with these types of experiences are normally represented and stored in what Bucci (1985) calls the "perceptual channels." In Luria's conceptualizations (1973), this information is organized primarily by the primary functional unit of the brain but also with the involvement of the secondary functional unit as well. They become part of a comprehensive memory matrix against which other data are assessed and processed. It is in this context that we acquire a sense of ourselves and our connection to the world as our psychic structures are formed (as depicted in Figure 5.5). These are the data that Winnicott (1965), Sullivan

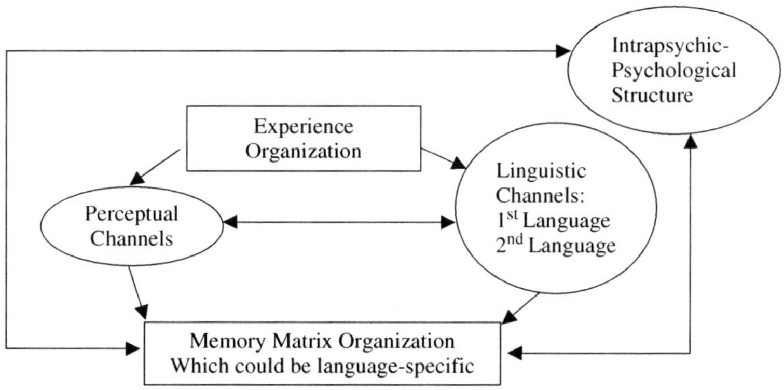

FIGURE 5.5. Psychic organization in a bilingual context.

(1953), and Kohut (1977) found to be so crucial for the development of psychic formation and that become ingrained in the individual's self-representation.

When verbal codification is used to mediate these experiences, the "linguistic channel" becomes the mode of memory representation. Words learned in that context become a powerful symbolic means to organize these experiences. The texture of these experiences and memories, the quality of the introjects, and identifications thus developed may then become more closely connected to that specific language function (the mother tongue), although some of the experiences may have been organized at the nonverbal level (Locke, 1994).

Although many learning situations rely heavily on verbal expression, it is clear that the full memory of the specific experience can be said to be possible when the individual is able to connect with the aspects of experience that are organized at the perceptual channel. Depending on the extent to which linguistic approximation is found for information organized along the perceptual channel, memories associated with these experiences can be, in part, verbally retrieved. I say in part because the extent of approximation depends on the quality of what Bucci (1985) called "referential activity," which varies between individuals "as a matter of competence, and may vary within an individual over time as a function of external context or inner state" (p. 589).

In the case of bilinguals, I suggest that the individual's relationship to his or her languages may also determine the mode and extent to which these memories may be accessed linguistically. As discussed earlier, bilinguals do develop different linguistic organizations depending on the level of linguistic proficiency and on the way the languages are learned (Ervin & Osgood, 1954). We discussed earlier that when the individual learns and becomes proficient in a second language later in life, the two languages remain relatively separately organized in the brain, each with its own phonemic, syntactic, symbolic, ideational components, and memory structure. A "coordinate linguistic organization" is thus said to have taken place. A "compound bilingual organization" is said to have taken place when the languages are learned at the same time, spoken by the same people, and refer to the same experiences (Ervin & Osgood, 1954; Javier & Marcos, 1989). Both languages are assumed to be organized along a common unitary linguistic structure.

A coordinate linguistic organization, by definition, implies that the two languages remain relatively independent from one another, or what has been called the "language independence phenomenon" (Javier & Marcos, 1989; Marcos & Alpert, 1976), while compound linguistic organization allows for more interplay between or among the languages. That this is the case was amply demonstrated by previously discussed psycholinguistic works of Lambert (1972), Ervin (1963), Marcos and Alpert (1976), Ojemann and Whitaker (1978), Albert and Obler (1978), and my own work (Javier, 1995; Javier & Marcos, 1989). Findings from these investigations suggest that even in the case of a compound bilingual organization, most individuals develop a coordinate bilingual organization for some of their experiences while simultaneously developing a compound organization for others.

Part of the reason for this has to do with the specific semantic, phonemic, and grammatical structures of the languages involved, which make a one-to-one relationship between or among the languages impossible. Some languages, for instance, may even lack certain concepts altogether or have specific concepts much more developed than others, as in the case of the Eskimos referred to earlier whose concepts for "snow" surpass the concepts of those speaking other languages. According to Kolers' (1968) study discussed earlier, however, it is more likely that concepts related to affective state (love, hate, frustration) and abstract formulations (e.g., freedom, country) may remain more language-specific than concepts related to concrete experiences. This may explain how some bilinguals may find it easier to curse in one language and difficult to do so in another, or may find that their associations to dream material can be easier and more fluid in one language, though not necessarily the language of the dream. This was the case of the patient described in a recent presentation by Schlachet and Aragno (1994) who was unable to associate to the "bear" of his dream; his associative process became liberated when translation into the Spanish "*oso*" was made, which was associated with conflictual memories of an abusive father.

From this perspective, we can see how the accessibility of memory developed in relation to one of the languages depends on the nature and quality of the patient's linguistic organization, the extent of contextual cues in the environment, and the individual's emotional organization (Riccio, et al., 1994). For Schrauf (2000), memories from any period of life may be accessed and retrieved or reconstructed from within the second language but that retrieval is not the same in both languages. According to him, childhood memories, for instance, when retrieved in the mother tongue, "may be more numerous, more detailed, more emotional or more vibrant than when retrieved in the second language" (p. 388). Thus, it is the language of the experience that determines the extent and meaningfulness of the recollection.

Following Weingartner's conceptualization (1978) and my own conceptualization regarding the nature of repression in bilinguals (1996), he suggests that remembering could be a function of the extent to which the "language spoken (a qualitative "state") at the time of retrieval matches the language spoken (another qualitative "state") at the time of memory encoding." That is, the extent to which the condition that characterized the initial processing of the experience can be successfully recreated (state-dependent learning) at the time of the retrieval. It is a cognitive perspective that emphasizes the importance of context in learning and memory retrieval.

The other factor that affects memory retrieval discussed by Schrauf (2000) has to do more with the individual self-concept that develops in the context of his or her language development. It is based on his belief that when a bilingual speaks one or the other of his or her languages, it activates a "language-specific self" that acts as filter through which memories are both encoded and retrieved. Thus "memories of childhood events are 'filtered through' a socioculturally constituted, linguistically mediated, *first*-language self... Memories for recent events, meanwhile, are 'filtered through' a socioculturally constituted, linguistically mediated, *second*-language self..." (p. 388). This explanation emphasizes the role of the self-representation, or psychic organization, in language function, in terms of both its development and its role in guiding the individual's cognitive and emotional functioning.

A remaining question is the issue of how experience that has occurred at the prelinguistic level can be organized and can become accessible linguistically. That is, how are we to have access to the kinds of experiences that are organized around nonverbal representations and thus become lodged in a "perceptual mode" of memory organization? Are we to assume, in keeping with previous comments, that the language that develops closer in proximity to these experiences will be the language of preference to access memories associated with these experiences? If this is the case, however, how are we to understand the role of intrapsychic structure in language development that Buxbaum (1949), Greenson (1950), Krapf (1955), Marcos (1976), Perez-Foster (1992), and Javier (1989, 1995, 1996) have amply discussed in previous writings in which it is the described the way intrapsychic dynamic linked to the material under consideration will determine the nature and extent of its accessibility?

What I am saying here is that memory accessibility is complicated under the best of circumstances and even more so in the case of bilinguals. We need to consider, among other things, the interplay of intrapsychic structure and language representation and how language can become subservient to emotional (psychic) demands, in addition to the normal linguistic complications in memory function (Schrauf, 2000). Moreover, we also need to consider the possibility that an experience that is not accessible in one language may be accessible in another and hence the concept of the inaccessibility of information as a result of the operation of a psychological mechanism, such as repression, may not apply (Javier, 1995).

I suspect that all our experiences are organized along sensory–perceptual and linguistic channels to various degrees (along a dual linguistic channel in the case of a bilingual) and that personal (intrapsychic/unconscious) forces become increasingly more influential with regard to how these experiences are ultimately organized along these channels, as suggested in Figure 5.5. That psychological (intrapsychic) structure can affect the perceptual channel processing has been demonstrated by patients whose ability to perceive and feel is distorted due to anxiety. In extreme cases, it can be seen in patients suffering from hysterical blindness, pseudocyesis, paralysis, sexual dysfunction, and dyspnea (Freud, 1896). Examples of the extent to which language function can be affected by intrapsychic conflict can be seen in patients suffering from speech disturbances due to anxiety and unconscious conflicts, as described by Greenson (1950) and Buxbaum (1949). The extent to which the different channels involved in organizing an experience shown in Figure 5.5 may ultimately represent different degrees of accessibility for memories connected to these personal experiences; and the extent to which having two linguistic codes may facilitate as much as hinder accessibility of important memories, suggest that the phenomenon of repression may have a very different quality when applied to a bilingual individual.

Investigation of Bilingual Personal Memory

Those interested in investigating more systematically and under more control conditions how memory of emotional import (such as personal memory or autobiographical memory, referred to above) is coded linguistically in bilingual individuals have been frustrated by the way these types of memories are normally investigated. Indeed, investigation of bilingual memory has followed traditional lines of investigating this phenomenon, focusing, for the most part, on the assessment of linguistic representational processing of experiences (Kolers & Paradis, 1980), and assuming that word association tasks (Davis & Wertheimer, 1967; Kolers, 1963), list-learning tasks (Goggin & Wickens, 1971; Lambert, Ignatow, & Krauthamier, 1968), and reading comprehension tasks (Macnamara & Kushnir, 1971) would give an accurate description of the kinds of bilingual memories possible, including personal memories, and has attempted, in this context, to provide a characterization of the bilingual memory system. These studies have emphasized primary nonpersonal memory phenomena and thus leaving us without sufficient information to advance our understanding of memory of a more personal nature. We are left, then, with the question as to the best way to examine these types of memories in all their complexity.

In an article published in the *American Psychologist*, Banaji and Crowder (1989) suggested that only traditional (laboratory) approaches to the study of human memory have any scientific value. These authors strongly criticized investigations that incorporate naturalistic methodology for the examination of the everyday personal memory. In their view, the fact that the main thrust of naturalistic approaches is the examination of the phenomena in their natural condition means that they “largely abandon the opportunities for analytic control of the learning and test condition . . .” (p. 1186). They claim that naturalistic studies compromise the generalization and external validity power of the findings.

Banaji and Crowder’s view is troublesome since it attempts to reduce and simplify a process that is, by its very nature, quite complex. Their suggestions that memory of personal events is best studied through the episodic memory research approach has been criticized by other authors as naïve and simplistic (Ceci & Bronfenbrenner, 1991; Conway, 1991). One of the problems is that in episodic memory research all extraneous variables are controlled and variables of interest are closely manipulated and hence not conducive to an examination of memory phenomena of a personal nature in their natural condition (Conway, 1991). The experimental task, usually words in a word list, is devoid of personal meaning and, thus, only memory for microfeatures of an event can be assessed.

By contrast, autobiographical memory research starts from the premise that the best way to investigate the phenomenon is the one that allows to capture the richness of personal meaningful memory in a controlled naturalistic environment, without any attempts to control or restrict meaning (Conway, 1990a, b, 1991). Memories of personal events presuppose a meaningful emotional connection with events usually including, but not limited to, experiences accumulated over time. These experiences provide an organizing framework for the individual's life and result in autobiographical memory or "memory for information related to the self" (Brewer, 1986, p. 33). These memories are more likely to be well-remembered because they are usually unique, unexpected, emotionally provoking, and/or idiosyncratically meaningful. In fact, the more an individual is able to make affective connection with a task to be remembered, including nonsense lists, the more likely that the specific memory under consideration will be successfully retrieved.

The nature and extent to which memory of personal events are linguistically organized and retrieved in bilinguals was demonstrated experimentally (Javier et al., 1993) and in clinical observations (Buxbaun, 1949; Greenson, 1950; Javier, 1995, 1996; Marcos, 1976; Perez-Foster, 1992, 1996). In the study by Javier and associates, for instance, on the basis of a free-association methodology suggested by Bucci and Freedman (1978, 1981) and Bucci (1982, 1985), a coordinate bilingual group with equal proficiency in both languages was asked to communicate a personal (dramatic) experience in the same language that they were using when the event occurred. At a later point, they were asked, unexpectedly, to communicate the same experience in the other language. The linguistic order of the narrative was counterbalanced to control for possible language effect. The production in both languages was subjected to a careful and elaborate linguistic analysis with regard to the quality of the idea and thought units (Chafe, 1980). Our findings suggest that the immediacy of the context in which the verbal interaction occurs and the length of the subject's linguistic experience in that context may both influence the extent to which a language will serve as a reference point for a specific experience. It was found that the nature and quality of these memories differed significantly in both languages. For instance, subjects tended to provide a richer detailed and evocative rendition of an experience in one language and reduce the same experience to a functional and laconic production in the other language.

This was the case regardless of the language of the experience, suggesting that for a bilingual with coordinate linguistic organization, the language of the experience or where the specific memory is more meaningfully encoded may not be necessarily the primary language.

This is an important finding that is at the very center of an often-held belief that the individual's first language is the language of the affect. Our finding suggests that both languages are used to code affect and depending upon the specific content of concern, one or the other language may be closer to affective material. Of course, when we are dealing with early experiences that developed in connection with the first language, then emotions connected to those experiences are expected to be more accessible in the first language. Similarly, emotions connected with experiences that developed in the context of the second language are expected to be more accessible in the second language.

Concluding Thoughts

In summary, the brain is a complex system where memories of experiences are progressively organized to allow the organism to respond to the demands of the external and internal environments. Memory allows the individual to remember and organize events and experiences of various kinds through his or her life cycle. It allows the individual to organize and categorize information received from different internal and external sources. There are different kinds of memories possible, such as memory for places, for objects, events, people (Baddeley, 1991; Cohen, 1991; Riccio et al., 1994) and, as demonstrated, there are different parts of the brain involved in the development of these memories (Locke, 1994; Luria, 1973, 1981). Language function is intimately involved in these memory organizations and allows for much more sophisticated storage/retrieval of human experiences and hence our tendency to focus on language expression to assess and treat our patients. Because of the unique role of language in all mental processes, in the course of the chapter I focused my attention on a discussion of the nature of the bilingual memory and the factors affecting its accessibility. Special emphasis was made on a discussion of the way affects are linguistically codified and made accessible. We recognize that the nature of the individual bilingualism and his or her level of proficiency and linguistic organization have major implications on the nature and extent of accessibility and the quality and accuracy of assessment of cognitive and emotional processes in bilinguals.

Take, for instance, the study reported by Marcos and associates (1973). These authors interviewed ten schizophrenic patients in the patient's first language (Spanish) and also in the second language (English). The videotape recordings of these interviews were evaluated independently by four psychiatrists (two Spanish-speaking and two English-speaking), utilizing the brief psychiatric rating scale. The two Spanish-speaking psychiatrists evaluated the Spanish interview, while the two native English-speaking psychiatrists evaluated the English interview. The findings indicated that the level of pathology was found to be much higher in English than in Spanish. In fact, of the 18 scales of the Brief Psychiatric Rating Scales, six were most affected by the language of the interview (e.g., tension, depressed mood, hostility, anxiety, emotional withdrawal, and somatic concern.). In explaining the "affective detachment" observed in these patients when interviewed in English, Marcos (1976) stated that "the information-processing mechanism involved in the speaking of the language which is not the primary tongue may function as an impediment to the emotional expression and affective involvement of the person" (p. 552).

Another pertinent study is the one by Sollee (1963) and reviewed by Schneider (1981). Reportedly, Sollee subjected two symmetrical (coordinate) bilingual groups of children to a series of taboo and neutral words in both of the bilinguals' languages. The tachistoscopic recognition thresholds of these words were then measured. One of the bilingual groups learned the Philippine language "Tagalog" at home and English at a later period, while the reverse was true for the other group. Sollee found that taboo words in the mother tongue generated more anxiety than taboo words in the second language. This was evident by the higher tachistoscopic recognition thresholds to taboo words in the first language. The threshold scores for the taboo words in both languages were higher than for the neutral words.

Similar findings were reported by Gonzalez-Reigosa (1976) who studied the level of anxiety generated by a group of taboo words in both languages of a group of bilinguals. Utilizing the Spielberger State-Trait Anxiety Inventory to measure levels of anxiety, he found that saying taboo words in the mother tongue aroused more anxiety than saying such taboo words in the language acquired late in life. In explaining the individual's anxiety reaction to taboo words, Greenson (1950) suggests that "obscene words force the listener to a regressive hallucinatory reexperience of memory pictures" and as "these words... remain the living bearers of unresolved conflicts," their usage puts the individual in contact with emotions attached to these conflicts (p. 20).

However, there are a number of experiences that the individual goes through as he or she goes from one developmental stage to another, from one situation to another (such as home, school, employment), or in interactions with one or another person (e.g., parents, teachers, friends). We can then assume that the emotions associated with these experiences would become closely associated with the language utilized for those experiences. Or, stated differently, the emotions associated with the second language may correspond to psychological stages in the individual that are different from the stages associated with the first language. If an individual learns the second language during adolescence and utilizes it, for example, only in school, then emotions associated with the school experience are expected to be more powerfully communicated in the second language. Thus, it is not that the second language carries less emotional import but that the emotional contents associated with the second language are of a different nature.

6
Communication Through Interpreters

A natural outcome of a multilingual community is the fact that the need for translation/interpretation of information becomes inevitable. This is particularly the case when the languages spoken in the specific community are not known equally by all the members of that community. I discussed in the previous chapters the thousands of languages spoken in the world and how members of these different linguistic communities are immigrating to different countries (such as Europe and the United States and Canada) in search of better living conditions (Lehrer & Sloan, 2005). The political fluidity in many countries is likely to intensify this phenomenon even further in the years ahead. Thus, the possibility for distortion in the communication becomes even more likely as the linguistic community become more numerous and diverse.

Do we know enough about what system is being utilized by the military in Afghanistan and Iraq to bridge the communication between serving men from the United States and women and the citizens of these Arab-speaking countries? The report is that crash courses are precipitously organized to provide them with simple phrases and then they rely heavily on interpreters. Although we recognize the merit of deciding to use interpreters to bridge the communication between and among individuals who need to communicate with one another but who do not have the necessary knowledge of each other's languages, it could be a very dangerous endeavor, indeed. This is particularly the case when there is an assumption of adequate communication of the intended message, and actions are then taken based upon that communication (i.e., deciding to shoot someone because of the apparent refusal to follow a directive from the military). A good translation is hard and can only be said to have been accomplished when the content of the communication, including the speaker's intention, and the paralinguistic components of the message are also translated and interpreted in the target language, including the specific linguistic and paralinguistic characteristics of the specific linguistic community of the listener.

To say that interpretation is a complicated process is an understatement considering the complexity of the whole process of communication even in the monolingual condition described in Chapter 2 (Table 2.1). Thus, it is not surprising that complication in the communication could occur especially when untrained interpreters are involved in the interpretation process. The fact of the matter is that interpreters are now required to be routinely incorporated as part of the evaluation and treatment process in many metropolitan hospitals in

New York City and are essential ingredients in places like the United Nations. Even major telecommunication industries, such as AT&T, maintain a language bank of interpreters, covering a variety of languages that are available to provide linguistic services.

It is not unusual, however, that in response to the shortage of bilingual/bicultural professionals, many institutions tend to rely on untrained interpreters – such as janitors, clerical helpers, other professionals, and even patients or relatives of patients – to transmit information between and among different parties (Marcos, 1989; Vazquez & Javier, 1991). Although practical considerations are usually cited as the reason for this occurrence, such a practice represents a tremendous danger to the process of communication, with potentially disastrous effects. It certainly puts in doubt the accuracy of the evaluation and intervention given to these patients. An example of this dangerous practice was discussed by Nina Bernstein in her recent article in the *New York Times* (April 21, 2005) entitled "Language Barrier Called Health Hazard in ER." In this article she referred to a case of a woman who had to rely on her English-speaking Korean cabdriver to translate a doctor's direction for treating her 11-year-old son. She also referred to another case of doctors communicating with a construction worker, through his 7-year-old cousin, that he needed an amputation, only to receive from the child that he was not sure if the doctors said toe or foot. In a previous publication (Vazquez & Javier, 1991) we discussed a case similar to the one discussed by Bernstein (2005) whose symptoms of depression were minimized in the process of the translation by her 13-year-old nephew. In this case, a woman suffering from depression with a suicidal condition had to be psychiatrically evaluated through interpretation provided by the woman's nephew. On the way to the psychiatrist, the woman asked the nephew to promise her that he will make sure that she was not taken to the hospital. This woman's depressive condition was precipitated by the death of her mother in the country of origin whose funeral she could not attend because of her illegal status in this country. Thus, when responding to the psychiatrist's questions she stated that she had been feeling depressed, was crying, was unable to eat and sleep, was thinking constantly about her mother, and that she has been struggling to cope. The nephew's rendition of that communication was that her aunt was not feeling well but that she is struggling and that she was okay.

There were serious mistakes made in this transaction that were amply discussed in that paper, but what I wanted to emphasize here is that the personal agendas of the individuals involved in the communication will determine and influence the final product, especially in the case of untrained interpreters. The fact that such a practice is still maintained in spite of its potentially serious implications reinforces the need to encourage further discussion of the complexity inherent in the whole process of communication and how the intended communication can be so easily derailed when untrained interpreters are used. In this chapter we will address further the crucial role played by interpreters and will outline briefly the complex nature of the interpretation process, making specific references to common errors normally found in interpretation.

Communication Process

Communication between two individuals in a monolingual condition involves the process of transmitting (decoding and encoding), verbally and nonverbally, different perceptions, experiences of various kinds, beliefs, thought processes, worldviews, individual and group identities, specific cultural characteristics, as well as the affective components associated with these perceptions, experiences, beliefs, and thoughts (Dana, 1993; Vazquez & Javier, 1991). When an individual is successful in communicating all these aspects and when the listener is able to decipher the code, a successful communication is assumed to have occurred. The height of this experience is seen when the individual attempting to communicate feels "understood" and experiences the listener as "receptive."

When the communication occurs between individuals whose worlds have developed in different geographical, cultural, and linguistic contexts (Ervin, 1963; Whorf, 1956), as in the case of the bilingual experience, it is even more difficult to gauge accurately what is being communicated. The possibility for misconception, therefore, depends on the level of proximity of the personal, cultural, and linguistic histories of the individuals involved in the communication. When such histories are too diverse, the possibilities for misunderstandings and gaps in the communication are even greater (Dale, 1972). This communication gap, however, can be reduced provided that there is an active attempt on the part of the participants in the communication to have better appreciation, respectful awareness, acceptance, and sensitivity not only at the linguistic level but also at the cultural, political, socioeconomic levels between and among those involved. Dana (1993) suggested in this regard that the main obstacle to understanding in the multicultural context is the multiplicity of belief systems or worldviews that are likely to collide the more diverse they are. What is required is the recognition that the speaker and the listener are equally important to the successful outcome of the communication. It requires a suspension of value judgments and preconceived notions on the part of both the speaker and the listener, so that the full power of the intended communication is received unaltered.

This nonjudgmental attitude has been described in the psychoanalytic literature as "evenly suspended attention" (Freud, 1912), "listening with a third ear" (Reik, 1958) and that was amply described by Freedman (1983) in his article "On Psychoanalytic Listening." Freedman was able to describe the complexity inherent in the listening process and identify specific components (e.g., receiving and restructuring phases) involved in a successful listening. When one is in the receiving phase, there is an openness to the intent of the other and a receptiveness to the multiple alternatives being communicated, with less need to objectify and create symbolic representation of the message. That is, attention remains open and uncompromised, allowing for multiple possibilities to occur. By contrast, during the restructuring phase, the emphasis is on a narrowing of the attention and a reduction of the possibilities for the purpose of reaching an objectification of the message and a consolidation of the symbolic representation of the message.

This way of listening to the information allows not-easily-understood data to become part of the information bank that can then influence the nature of the interaction. A complication in any of these different components in the listening process can result in distortions in the communication, which are then multiplied tenfold when a multilingual condition is involved.

Thus, monolingual communication or communication between and among bilinguals with comparable proficiency in their languages requires some level of translation but such a process does not involve a third person as mediator. In the interpretation process, on the other hand, three individuals are involved in the communication process, one functioning as the mediator of the communication between the two main actors.

Components of Communication

Thus, recognizing that the need for interpretation of a message is not unique to a multilingual community but occurs even in a monolingual, we can distinguish four basic components that are present in any communication:

1. Speaker or sender of the message, with his or her attitudes and personal/cultural characteristics, belief systems, worldview, personal and group identities, encoding skills, and intentionality
2. The listener or receiver of the message, with his or her attitudes and personal/cultural characteristics, belief systems, worldview, personal and group identities, decoding skills, and intentionality
3. Message to be communicated
4. Channel(s) used for the transmission of the message (Keltner, 1970; Figure 6.1).

Thus, implied in Figure 6.1 is the fact that the process of interpretation is in operation in the normal process of communication even between and among individuals who, although speaking apparently the same language, may have come from different experiences and geographical contexts. Consider, for

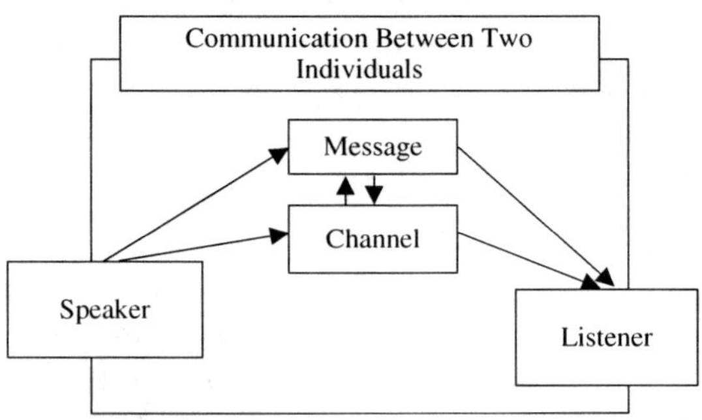

FIGURE 6.1. Interpretation process.

instance, the English language spoken by someone coming from the South, Midwest, or Northeast of the United States or coming from England or Jamaica. Or Spanish spoken by someone from South America, Central America, the Caribbean, or Spain. Each of these regions carries its own characteristics and flavor that are unique to the region and are transmitted in specific linguistic modes (Javier & Camacho-Gingerich, 2004). Hence, we find ourselves constantly needing to translate and rework specific information to ensure that we are getting the intended meaning even in a monolingual condition.

I still remember my experience in Venezuela, standing with a group of youngsters from that country and other Latin American countries and observing a group of nuns who were walking up the mountain through a narrow street and were forced to press their bodies against the edge of the mountain whenever a vehicle approached too close to them for fear of being hurt. At one point, a car stopped and invited them to get in, to which someone from Latin America said rather expressively, "*miren, las monjas están cogiendo una bola*," to mean "look, the nuns are taking a ride" in the country of origin of the speaker. However, it raised a few eyebrows because, for some of the listeners, it meant something that should not be used in reference to a respectful/religious person. It meant that the nuns are grabbing the male genitalia. The same group of youngsters again found themselves in another embarrassing situation when one of them referred to a large beautiful and multicolor parrot as "*cuca*" and used "*bellaco*" to refer to someone who is mischievous (or a teaser) while in the midst of a social gathering with prominent individuals. These concepts in that country refer to a woman's genitalia and to someone who is sexually promiscuous, respectively.

Consider a more subtle example that could happen when two different cultural styles of communication are maintained, although the language appears to be the same, with devastating effect. This occurred between two individuals in high positions at an academic institution where at one time the atmosphere became extremely charged with mutual accusations of distrust because, according to one, "you never tell me straight what you think or what should happen" or "you are rude and insulting in your communication and always violate the confidential nature of what is discussed," according to the other. Part of the complaint is that there is a feeling that what one takes as a sign of a decision having being reached ("I see what you are saying"), the other sees it as only showing respect for that point of view, not wanting to contradict it in public. Another complaint by one of these individuals was that the communication from the other is not genuine because, although it appears to be friendly at times, it is expected that the other will just comply with specific requests, requiring of this individual complete submission and relinquishment of any decision-making position. The result is that this individual then experiences the interaction between them as threatening and thus with the need to erect a defensive attitude against the other. To the extent to which the need to protect (a self or a position) becomes more prevalent in the interaction, the communication between these two individuals will be equally affected. Refusing to meet face to face, they now use e-mails as a mode of communication. But since the issue complicating the communication between these individuals is partly due to different cultural styles of communication, misinterpretation of the content and intention of the communication still occurs.

The point of this section was to emphasize the importance of keeping in mind that there are too many things that can complicate the communication even in a monolingual context and that this is even more so when more than one language is involved. In the next section, we will focus our attention on describing more specifically the interpretation process that, by definition, requires three individuals, one functioning as the mediator of the communication between the two main actors. The process of interpretation from one language to another is not just a linguistic exercise but requires an appropriate knowledge and appreciation of the culture, geographical characteristics, sociopolitical and sociolinguistic realities, regionalism, educational background as well as the logic systems of interpersonal communications of both the speaker and the receiver of the message. That is, it requires a process of interpretative transposition of the message. This allows the intended meaning of the communication to have a better chance to retain its accuracy.

Distinguishing Characteristics of Interpretation versus Translation Process

The process of interpretation refers to a very specific process that is often confused with that of translation. A definition distinguishing these terms is, thus, relevant here. In this chapter, we will use the concept of interpretation to refer to the process of communicating orally across linguistic/cultural barriers (Arjona, 1977). It does not involve a literal linguistic transposition of the message, but the oral translation of the intended meaning. A translation, on the other hand, is the communication of information from one language to another in written form. According to Arjona (1977), it refers to the interlingual, sociolinguistic, cultural transfer of any message from one individual to another through various modes of written, oral, or mechanical means or combination thereof. It is a specialized discipline of academic studies. According to Johnson (2000), translation requires movement among different levels of mental representation. When one is translating (and I would venture to say even when one is interpreting) from language A to language B, it is required that the translator mentally move from the linguistic-representational level of A to the logological structure level of word reference (abstract aspect of language, the metalinguistic characteristics), to the infralogical level (concrete physical experience) for the precise sense in the current context. According to Johnson, processing must then move back to the logological level of meaning and finally to the linguistic-structural level of language B.

As described in Chapter 2, infralogical structures are particular-experiential structures or structures of the life world with strong reference to the "first level of experience organization" or experience related to the sensory–motor dimension (Figure 2.2). They are the substance of experience and represent actual objects or things in the environment. According to Johnson (2000), they also include internal representations for distal objects whether they are organized as prototypes, scripts, or schemas. These structures organize the world senses or the concrete physical experiences the child has with its immediate environment. Logological structures are said to be in place when the particular-experiential structures (infralogical structures) are encoded and organized into kinds (or classes, relations, or propositions). Logological structures are of a higher order than their infralogical referents, "they are genetic kinds that often represent common characteristics of the infralogical token structures from which they are constructively abstracted" (Johnson, 2000, p. 194). As we said earlier, they embody invariances across types of objects or situations and hence they are more abstract structures, higher level or meta-organizations and as such distinct from the infralogical structures that they can represent. Finally, linguistic structures encode invariances in the linguistic environments (e.g., lexical terms, grammatical relations) and are expected to mediate communication among humans.

Two different theories have been proposed to explain the interpretation process. One follows the Lexical Hypothesis Model while the other suggests that the process is best served by a Conceptual Mediation Hypothesis Model (Islam & Lane, 1994). If one believes that interpretation is only a process of finding links between lexical equivalents in the bilingual speakers' two languages, the lexical hypothesis is assumed to be in place. But if one maintains that in order for interpretation to be effective it has to engage conceptual structures shared by two lexicons, then the Conceptual Mediation Hypothesis is believed to be in operation.

Following a Conceptual Mediation paradigm, Islam and Lane (1994) explain the process of interpretation as follows:

> The interpreter proceeds initially as the monolingual listener would. The incoming string is segmented, parsed and transformed into nonlinguistic propositional representations at the conceptual level. Each proposition, in turn, modifies, expands, and otherwise alters an ongoing model of discourse. From this discourse model, a preverbal message is prepared for delivery to the target language system, which plans a grammatical target-language sentence just as if the proposition had originated with the interpreter. (p. 294)

Thus, the Conceptual Mediation Hypothesis gives a central role to comprehension, while the role of comprehension is less clear in the Lexical Hypothesis Model, although it may still be present.

Of great importance here is the clarification that fluency of language alone is not sufficient for the quality of interpretation and/or translation. It is also important to recognize that these processes are not automatic within individuals. In fact, it is actually believed that they require an innate ability (Grosjean, 1982). This notwithstanding, the complexity of the process of translation and interpretation skills as such can be developed through training (Acosta & Cristo,

1981; Arjona, 1977). A good interpreter is one who is able to render the original message into the necessary meaningful linguistic and paralinguistic symbols and codes of the listener's culture and language (Arjona, 1977). It is not surprising, from this perspective, that the interpretation provided by the unsophisticated and untrained interpreters, such as those routinely used by hospitals and clinics, are often fraught with many inaccuracies and distortions; hence, the question is whether you are communicating with your clients, especially when the interaction between the professional and the client is being mediated by an unsophisticated interpreter.

Challenges to Accurate Interpretation

The challenges to proper interpretation are enormous, including the fact that there are idioms, concepts, regionalisms whose translation from one language to another is almost impossible.

Consider, for instance, the following phrases in various languages derived from several sources, including from Fabbro, Gran, Baso, and Brava (1990):

- *Déjate de hablar pleplas/pendejadas* (stop talking nonsense)
- *En la casa del ahorcado no se habla de soga* (in the house of the hung one, you shouldn't mention rope)
- *A tontas y a locas* (in a helter-skelter way)
- *Hay que verlo para creerlo* (the proof is in the pudding)
- *Un chota, un soplón* (tattle tale . . .)
- *Por si las moscas* (just in case)
- A bird in the hand is worth two in the bush
- *Un pájaro en manos major que tres volando* (a bird in the hand is better than three in flight)
- That boy is as fit as a fiddle
- The early bird catches the worm
- *Para comida perdida barriga partida* (rather a stomachache than wasted food)
- Waste not want not
- An idle brain is the devil's workshop
- You can't teach an old dog new tricks
- Little wit in the head makes much work for the feet
- Every cloud has its silver lining
- *Sine-Qua-Non*
- *Un tapón de tráfico* (a traffic jam)
- *Gutta cavat lapidem* (so much the drop falls on a stone until it makes a hole)
- *La situazione era cosi difficile che non sapevo piu a che santo Votarmi* (the situation is so difficult that I do not know what saint to turn to)
- *E'difficile seguire il suo discurso perche salta sempre di palo en Frasca* (it is difficult to follow what you say or your discourse because you always jump from one thing to another)
- *Quando ascolti, devi fare attenzione a non prendere fischi per fiaschi* (things are not always what they seem)

Each of these phrases triggers specific images in the native speaker of these languages that the interpreter attempts to successfully bridge in order to render the communication as close as possible to the intended meaning. It is one of the most difficult challenges for any interpreter since idioms are impregnated with so much meaning and provide a unique linguistic flavor to the communication that can only be unlocked by someone familiar with the meaning. If the interpreter is not familiar with the specific linguistic way an intended meaning is coded, he or she is likely to rely on literal translation to bridge the communication, resulting in different mental images. Take, for instance, the idiom in English "a bird in hands is worth two in the bush;" in Spanish the same idiom is "un pajaro en manos es mejor que tres volando" (a bird in the hand is better than three in flight), which triggers a different mental image of birds flying rather than in the bush.

Another common obstacle to interpretation referred to in an earlier publication (Javier et al., 1998) is the one offered by an individual with a mental condition. Indeed, interpretation of the mental patient's verbalizations requires, in addition to the cultural and linguistic issues referred to above, knowledge of the professional jargon, specific concepts, including understanding of blocking, derailment, tangentiality, and other indicators of thought disorders or markers of psychopathology (Bellak & Faithorn, 1981; De Zulueta, 1984). Failure to do so could render the interview meaningless because the clinician will not be able to get an accurate picture of what the patient presents. For example, if a patient is blocking a thought or is using a convoluted structure of language, an untrained interpreter might construct the utterance to make sense and thus inject a personal meaning. Doing this type of reconstruction for the patient distorts and minimizes the actual pathology suffered by the patient and the clinician is left with a sanitized version of the patient's accurate communication. Similar distortion can also occur when the interpreter misconstrues the patient's verbalizations as more bizarre than what is experienced by others more familiar with the patient's cultural and linguistic background.

Regarding the role of culture in the interpretation process, it is important to clarify a common confusion. It is normally assumed that a bilingual person is automatically bicultural and a monolingual individual is automatically monocultural. Such confusion could not be further from the truth. This can easily be demonstrated in the case of French-speaking Britons or English-speaking Scots who are bicultural while remaining monolingual (Grosjean, 1982). In the United States we also find many English-speaking native Americans and second and third generation immigrants who share more than one culture, but only speak one language, English. This suggests the importance of accurately determining the cultural and linguistic characteristics of the individuals involved in the communication without making assumptions based on linguistic or cultural characteristics alone. This issue is at the very core of the assumed similarities within the different ethnic groups (e.g., Blacks, Latin American individuals, Asians coming from different geographical locations) and calls for an appreciation of the ways the similarities and differences among these individuals may impact on their linguistic and psychological behaviors.

Methods of Interpretation

The complexity of the interpretation process notwithstanding, distortions of communication can be greatly minimized when interpreters are properly selected and trained (Acosta & Cristo, 1981). Two main methods of interpretation have been identified in the literature: Simultaneous and Consecutive Interpretations. Of the two, Namy (1977), Arjona (1977), and Longley (1977) suggest that the simultaneous interpretation is the best method to apprehend and communicate the message in its plenitude. During this process, the interpreter renders the interpretation of the material concurrently or in very close proximity to the speaker's verbalization. It does not give much room for the interpreter to inject personal meaning or to evaluate the nature of the message.

Consecutive interpretation, on the other hand, lends itself to much more distortion of the message because the interpreter provides the interpretation after the speaker has completed part of or the whole message. Thus, the possibility for the injection of personal meaning and reorganization of the message is greatly enhanced. Implied in this categorization is the idea that, when dealing with a psychiatric condition, simultaneous interpretation provides the best condition when non-English-speaking patients have to be evaluated/treated by a monolingual English-speaking professional.

It is not within the scope of this chapter to provide a detailed description of, or an endorsement of, a specific interpretation method. It suffices to say at this point, however, that the simultaneous interpretation method was found to be effective in a pilot study conducted by Luis Marcos and Palma Valverde (personal communication). According to Namy, Arjona, and Longley, simultaneous interpretation allows the speaker the optimal access to the verbal and nonverbal aspects of the communication more directly and clearly (e.g., body language, tone of voice) in a way not provided by the other method. This is the case because the simultaneous interpretation method requires the interpreter to be physically positioned unobtrusively outside the visual field of the individuals involved in the communication (i.e., behind or at least by the side of the patient) as shown in Figure 6.2.

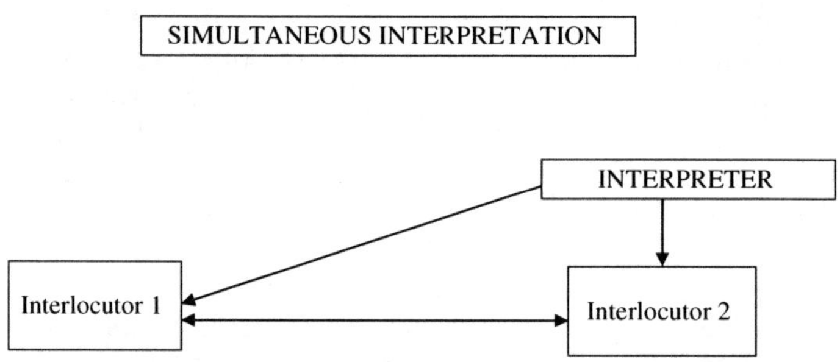

FIGURE 6.2. Simultaneous interpretation.

A successful interpreter is the one who functions solely as a "vessel" or a "conduit" of the communication between or among individuals without any personal intrusion and contamination. In this context, all that the interpreter does is to receive the message and provide a direct interpretation of that message by placing it in the cultural and linguistic context of the listener so that the intended meaning of the message is preserved.

In this method of communication the speaker directs his or her comments or questions directly to the interlocutor as if able to communicate directly with one another without assistance. Thus, in the case of the patient referred to earlier with a suicidal condition, the questions would have been:

- Tell me how can I help you?
- How have you been feeling?
- Have you been able to sleep or eat over the last week or so?

Rather the questions were directed to the nephew, and thus keeping him in the middle of the communication field and visually the focus of the interaction, as follows:

- Would you ask your aunt how I can help her?
- How has she been feeling?
- Has she been able to sleep or eat over the last week or so?

Training of Interpreters

A typical training for individuals interested in becoming proficient interpreters in a psychiatric setting normally includes role-playing on the following:

- The actual interpretation process
- The listening process
- Adequate facial and bodily movements.

There is also an intensive exposure to information on the following:

- The cultural, linguistic, and sociopolitical characteristics of the speaker
- The cultural, linguistic, and sociopolitical characteristics of the listener
- Typical concepts likely to emerge in the transaction (medical/psychiatric/legal/country specific).

In this regard, attention is given to the individual's accuracy of the interpretation, language proficiency, vocabulary usage, and recognition of terminology in the languages involved in the interpretation (Namy, 1977). That is, in order for the interpretation process to be effective, the interpreter is expected to be trained and to maintain proficiency in the specific content to be interpreted and hence it cannot be a fly-by-night operation or any able body used for the interpretation.

Common Errors

There are many ways in which an interpreter can render a message inaccurate and confusing (Marcos, 1989). The errors referred to here usually occur when an interpreter takes shortcuts or "literary liberty" because of a lack of familiarity with specific concepts, colloquial regionalism, slang, for lack of appreciation of the importance of accurate interpretation or for just lack of interest. The lack of interest may be particularly present in the case of unwilling interpreters who may experience interpreting as an additional burden to their already arduous job. In fact, in hospital situations where the demands for bilingual/bicultural professionals cannot be met, there is a tendency to rely on the few professionals with bilingual/bicultural backgrounds as well paraprofessionals and support staff. This, in turn, may contribute to an early burnout syndrome for these individuals.

In the following paragraphs I will utilize a series of linguistic transactions described in a previous publication (Javier et al., 1998) to illustrate the most common errors observed with untrained interpreters because I found these examples to drive home the point in the simplest and most direct manner. My decision to use transactions that occurred in a psychiatric setting as an example of interpretation errors is not only because they successfully represent the typical mistakes often found in linguistic transactions with untrained interpreters, but because there is an additional factor that needs to be considered (i.e., possible distortion of communication/thinking due to pathology) and that tend to complicate the picture further.

I will use the symbols "C", "P", and "I" to refer to the clinician, patient, and interpreter, respectively. I will only focus on the five basis common errors earlier identified by Vazquez and Javier (1991) and by Javier and his associates (1998): omission, addition, condensation, substitution, and role exchange.

Omission

It refers to a process by which an interpreter may delete completely or partially a message sent by a speaker. Examples of this error can be seen in the following exchanges mediated through an interpreter between a patient and a clinician:

Exchange 1

C. Well, it seems to me that it is difficult for her to talk about the family and how everybody is feeling.

I. *El... tenemos la impresión de que le es un poco difícil hablar de la situación de la familia y cómo se está sintiendo con la familia.* (He... We have the impression that it is a little difficult for you to speak about the family situation and how you are feeling with the family.)

P. Aha! (not translated)

C. I noticed that she (patient) smiled, could she tell me why?

I. *El nota que se sonríe, ¿le puedes explicar por qué?* (He notices that you smile, would you explain why)

P. *Es que le estoy explicando lo de mis hijas.* (It is that I am explaining about my daughters).
I. She said something, I don't know if I should go on . . .

Exchange 2

C. OK and how is she feeling about that plan?
I. *¿Y qué usted opina sobre ese plan?* (and what do you think about the plan)
P. *Bueno, segun ella me dijo, que era para ayudarme a mi, para darme la misma receta, para ayudarme al tratamiento que me daba ella.*
No me acuerdo. (Well, according to what she – social worker – told me, it was to help me, to give me the same prescription, medication, to help me in the treatment she was providing for me. I don't remember).
I. OK she says basically it was to help her . . . to continue her medication and to help her with the housing problem.

Exchange 3

C. Yes, were things ever different between her and her son?
I. *¿Usted, en algun momento, ha tenido una relación distinta con su hijo? ¿Las cosas eran distintas antes con él?* (You, at any moment have had a different relationship with your son? Were things different with him before?)
P. *¿Cómo?* (Not interpreted) (What?)
I. *¿Cómo ud. se llevaba con su hijo anteriormente?* (How did you get along with your son before?)
P. *Bien. Lo que lo hicieron así eran las malas amistades . . . esta vacio.* (Well, what made him like that were the bad companies. He is empty).
I. He wasn't really like that but . . . maybe he changes from his bad friends, wrong friends.
P. *Y no va a la escuela. No quiere ir a la escuela, no.* (he does not go to school, he refuses to go to school, no).
C. I see, so that must be very painful for her.
I. (not interpreted).

Although these three exchanges demonstrate different kinds of errors, the most prominent ones are errors of omission. In Exchange 1, for instance, the interpreter failed to relate to the clinician the patient's response to the question about the smile. Similarly, in Exchange 2, not only the patient's communication is condensed but the fact that the patient responded with "I don't remember" was never related to the clinician. In Exchange 3, the clinician's attempt to be empathic with the patient ("I see, so that must be very painful for her.") was not communicated to the patient. It is possible that the smile is inappropriate or that "I don't remember" is irrelevant or that the patient may ignore the clinician's attempt to be empathic; however, the clinician is not given all the information provided by the patient to make the evaluation and the patient is not provided with all the communication from the clinician, hence further diminishing the patient's chance to respond coherently.

Additions

This refers to an interpreter's tendency to include information not expressed by the speaker. It normally occurs in conjunction with a partial or complete omission of a message.

Exchange 4

C. Likewise, how her . . . could she tell me how she perceives the problem now, with her son?

I. *El ha leido sobre eso en su expediente, pero Usted puede decir un poco mas sobre ¿cómo estan los cosas con su hijo? Explicarle un poco más sobre su relación con su hijo.* (He has read about this in your record, but could you say more about how things are going with your son? Explain more about your relationship with your son)

P. *¿Qué es lo que pasó?* aha! (What happened? aha!) (not interpreted)

I. *Si, exacto.* (yes, exactly.)

P. *Pues, yo tengo un hijo de 14 años y me da muchos problemas por cuestión de malas amistades que tiene, este . . . ha cogido vicios con ellos y se busca problema en un hotel en que you vivo, este . . . .no respeta, no hace caso, en eso yo me he descontrolado los nervios.*

(Well, I have a 14-year-old son who gives me a great deal of trouble due to his bad company. he . . . .has picked up vices from them and gets himself in trouble at a hotel where I live, he . . . .does not show any respect, he does not pay attention, in that I have lost control of my nerves.)

I. She has a 14-year-old who has been giving her a hard time. He's been hanging around with wrong people. He's been now picking a lot of different kinds of vices, drugs, sounds like drug problems. She lives in a hotel and he's been giving problems there, getting into a lot of trouble.

In this exchange we can see how the interpreter's personal bias is added to the patient's message (". . . drugs, sounds like drug problems") while also condensing the patient's verbalization about her experience with her son. Her feeling that her son shows no respect and does not pay attention to her is not related to the clinician and hence the clinician may miss the interpersonal/cultural nature of the patient–son conflict. The impact of all of this tension on her ("I have lost control of my nerves") is not translated either, adding to the incomplete picture of the interaction.

Condensation

Condensation refers to an interpreter's tendency to simplify and explain a message sent by a speaker. It usually occurs when omission and addition has also taken place. It is clearly demonstrated in Exchange 2 when the patient's long response to the clinician's question is summarized with "she says basically . . ." Similarly, in Exchange 4 the same condensation process takes place with regard to the patient's experience with her son. As indicated earlier, the part of her message that is deleted, coupled with the elements added, can only contribute to an inaccurate appraisal of the patient's experience.

Substitutions

This error refers to an interpreter's tendency to replace concepts in a message sent by a speaker for the purpose of embellishing or condensing it. A change in the meaning of the message usually occurs. The errors resulting from the substituting aspect of the communication are, for the most part, related to the omission, addition, and condensation errors described above.

Consider the following exchange:

Exchange 5

C. Since you were started in the medicine, which was about 3 weeks, have you, eh, been, ah, experiencing anything unusual, like feeling that somebody is talking to you and there is nobody else there?

I. *Mientras estaba sobre la medicación, mientras estabas cogiendo la medicación, ¿tu oido "voices", te has sentido distinto, diferente, o de otra forma?* (While you were on the medication, while you were taking the medication, did you hear voices, or have you felt different... or in different way?).

P. No, *igual, siempre igual.* (No, the same, always the same)

I. He says, always the same.

C. What does that mean?

I. *¿Cómo, qué es igual?* (How, what is the same?)

P. *Bien, Bien!* (fine, fine!)

I. He says fine, fine!

In this exchange we can see that the patient's response is not to the clinician's question but to the interpreter's verbalization, resulting in confusion. In addition to condensation and addition errors, the interpreter substituted "somebody is talking to you and there is nobody else there" as "hearing voices" and "what does that mean?" for "what is the same?" The interpreter's verbalization "or felt different...?" resulted in the patient's "inappropriate" response ("always the same") to the clinician's question regarding the presence of "auditory hallucinations." Consequently, the issue of the auditory hallucinations could not be assessed.

Role Exchange

This error refers to the interpreter's tendency to take over the interaction and replace questions from the speaker with his or her own set of questions as if assuming the role of the clinician or the patient.

The following exchange demonstrates this error:

Exchange 6

C. And who . . . was any one else in the household?
P. No.
C. Do you have any other family besides your mother?
I. *¿Tiene other familia fuera de su mamà?*
P. *Sí, sí.* (yes, yes).
I. *¿Quienes?* (who?).
P. *Mis hermanos* (my brothers).
I. *¿Su hermanos? Cuánto?* (your brothers? How many?)
P. *Quince* (fifteen).
I. *¿Quince? ¿pero no viven todos juntos?* (fifteen? but, do you all live together?).
P. *No, en frente* (no, across the street from one another).

Although this particular exchange may not have serious consequences for the patient, consider what could happen in the situation involving an assessment of suicide or homicide potential. Since interpreters are not always knowledgeable of the crucial components necessary for such an assessment, they may fail to relate important information related by the patient to the clinician. Indeed, interpreters who make this kind of mistake usually tend to condense the message and include his or her view about the speaker's message. That was the issue in Exchange 4 when the interpreter indicated that ". . . sounds like drug problems," even though the patient never reported that. Such a situation was also amply described in an earlier paper (Vazques & Javier, 1991) and referred to earlier in this chapter in which the evaluation of a patient's level of suicidalogy was seriously compromised by a family member's inability to communicate to the clinician the patient's true psychiatric state. The family member failed to mention to the clinician the patient's depression or the fact that the patient was hearing her dead mother's voice.

Conclusion

The issues raised above regarding the negative consequence of communication errors cannot be sufficiently underlined. The different exchanges presented here attempted to demonstrate the deleterious effect of the different errors that an interpreter can make. They play a crucial role in rendering the communication between two interlocutors either clearly and accurately or in a confusing manner. The interpreter serves as a liaison, or a bridge, between two worlds, each with its own history, geography, belief systems, culture, language, and logic systems of interpersonal communication. Adequate interpretation poses a heavy burden for the interpreter, as the nature and quality of the interpretative activity may make a difference between life and death for some patients and for the public at large as well. In mental health, the nature and the quality of the treatment patients may receive could also be significantly impacted by poor interpretation. This is particularly the case with psychiatric patients who may have lost, partially or completely, the capacity to organize a fluid and chaotic subjective experience.

To avoid the complications resulting from inadequate interpretations provided by untrained interpreters, it is strongly recommended that individuals serving this role be properly trained (Acosta & Cristo, 1981, Arjona, 1977; Longley, 1977; Namy, 1977). Only in this manner will the intended meaning of the communication have a better chance to retain its accuracy. As shown earlier, individuals functioning as interpreters and lacking proper training tend to add, omit, condense, and/or substitute important information in the communication. Similarly, they tend to take on the role of the clinician and/or the patient (role exchange) and encourage the interaction between the patient and the clinician to remain detached and impersonal (e.g., using the third person pronoun, "The patient or the doctor said that...").

The deleterious impact of these types of errors on the evaluation of psychopathology was also assessed in a previous study by Marcos (1989). He concluded from this study that distortions in the communication could occur when the interpreters utilized have:

1. insufficient language competence and deficient interpretative skills;
2. insufficient psychiatric sophistication;
3. questionable attitude toward the patient and/or the clinician.

This issue of personal attitude is particularly problematic when using family members or other interpreters with strong personal views, as demonstrated by Marcos (1989) and by Vazquez and Javier (1991). For instance, Marcos described the reaction of a daughter who expressed strong negative feelings about the medication that the clinician had just prescribed and encouraged the mother not to take it. It is in these kinds of situations where pre–post interview meetings of the clinicians and interpreters are strongly encouraged. According to Marcos, these meetings should focus on a discussion of the goals of the evaluation, the focal areas to be assessed, and the interpreter's attitude regarding any aspects of the process.

There are different components and objectives in the training of interpreters. The goal of the training is ultimately to prepare better listeners who are able to render the original message into the necessary meaningful linguistic and paralinguistic symbols and codes of the listener's culture and language. The training of interpreters, however, for educational, medical, and mental health settings is only an interim and partial solution to a problem whose more adequate and ethical solution is the training and hiring of professionals with bilingual and bicultural backgrounds and with an appreciation of the participants' cultural and linguistic characteristics.

Finally, adding to the challenges in interpretation is the fact that interpreters are often faced with the almost insurmountable task of having to interpret communication from individuals whose idiosyncratic and peculiar linguistic behavior is not easily understood. Such a condition may contribute further to communication errors. In the case of medical and psychological evaluations or where a judge is attempting to determine guilt or innocence of an individual based upon what is being translated from the individual responses to questions from legal counsels, the prosecutor, and/or judge, the consequences of inaccurate translation could be quite enormous.

7 Issues in Assessing the Bilingual Individual

In this chapter, we will focus on the different factors/aspects that are likely to impact the assessment process of bilingual individuals, including those (such as personal motivation of the referring individual) that are difficult to quantify and evaluate because they could be rather subtle and not much research has been done on the subject. By "assessment" we refer to any condition where an evaluation of the bilingual individual's skills and cognitive/emotional status is performed. Thus, it includes formal and informal procedures, such as psychological tests, psychiatric and psychological interviews, psychosocial evaluations, vocational evaluations. These assessments could range from a brief to a more extensive process. But regardless of the length, the process tends to include a preliminary/initial fact-finding stage or initial assessment of the problem(s) and concludes with a recommendation stage, or a delineation of the specific ways to address the referral problem(s), including specific diagnosis, if requested as part of the referral question. Since each step of this process requires considerations of different factors that could influence the assessment outcome, we will now discuss these factors more specifically.

Personal Motivation/Specific Needs of the Referring Person

By the time a referral is made for an assessment of a bilingual individual a lot has usually gone on for the individual/child being referred to and in the mind of the person making the deferral. Usually an informal assessment of the situation has been made by the referring individual, which includes an appraisal of the specific issues of concern (e.g., behavior, learning difficulties), as well as his or her personal reaction. For instance, the teacher making a referral for assessment of a bilingual child may have made several complaints to the guidance counselor or the school administration delineating his or her frustration with the situation and may have made comments about the problematic student to other teachers. If the teacher making the referral has reached a high level of frustration and hopelessness with the situation, the referral is likely to read as follows: "I cannot have this child in my class, he or she is not learning, and/or the behavior is disrupting my class; he or she clearly does not fit in." A recommendation for a special class is likely to be included. In the case of a less frustrating situation, the teacher/guidance counselor may be more likely to focus on getting information about the child's unique issues affecting his or her ability to profit from the school environment and what they can do to address the situation.

Similar conditions may occur in the workplace or treatment condition where the employer/treating professional may feel frustrated with his or her difficulty in communicating or treating a linguistically diverse individual. It is here that the possibility for delegating such an individual to a less challenging work condition and the possibility of promotion becomes unlikely, although the individual may be otherwise very qualified or even overqualified for the position. When these individuals are in need of health and mental health services, a misdiagnosis and wrong focus in the treatment plan could occur, as delineated in the various chapters of this book and specifically in Chapter 6 on interpreters.

What I am referring to here is the need for those involved in assessing linguistically diverse individuals (but also important in any evaluation) to make sure that the personal motivation (personal bias) of the referring personnel does not inappropriately affect the objectivity of the assessment process and its recommendations. We can see the danger of this situation when a referral comes from someone who may enjoy a good reputation in their subject of expertise (e.g., biology, mathematics, social studies, laws, medicine, social work, psychology, dean of students) and is now insisting on an evaluation of the student's emotional state to determine if there is anything personally wrong or deficient with the student that can explain why he or she is failing and is unable to consider that the problem may be caused by something else. We can also see the same problem in operation when a professional is privately retained by an independent individual (a lawyer, legal system, parents looking for an independent evaluation) specifically to render an opinion, let's say, as part of a legal/educational procedure, and for which the professional is receiving its customary fee directly from these individuals. Sometimes the professional may feel, although not always verbalized, that there is an expectation of a specific outcome. Examples of these situations are of a lawyer/legal system that requests an evaluation of a bilingual child/individual as part of a litigation procedure because the child/individual may have been involved in an accident; or may have been exposed to lead intoxication; or as part of a child custody procedure in a contested divorce procedure; as part of an adoption procedure to determine appropriateness of fit between the child and the potential adoptive parents; or to determine insanity for a bilingual inmate convicted of murder but for whom an appropriate evaluation of his or her mental condition was not made, due to a language barrier. Another example is of a parent requesting a second opinion as part of a college application to support/repudiate a learning disability diagnosis.

Regardless of the reason(s) for the referral, the assessor should make it clear to the referring individual that information coming from various sources will be evaluated in the process of the assessment, in addition to the specific data derived from the tests administered, and that a recommendation will be made based on all the information gathered. In the case of an independent referral, it is strongly advised for the professional to require payment of fee prior to the end of the assessment process so that it makes it clear that the outcome of the assessment will be a function of the data gathered. The payment is for the time, not for the outcome of the assessment. Only by following this procedure, the assessment will likely remain free from the influence of the referring individual and hence the independence of the assessment process will be preserved.

An example of an inherent bias in the referring professional can be seen in the case of a university professor who brought a Chinese student for an assessment because the student was falling behind in most of his subjects, specially those requiring long written papers. Courses relying on formulas were less of a problem. The referring professional strong believed that the student's emotional problem, particularly depression, was the reason for his poor performance. He was living alone and was missing his family, which was still in China. There were no indications that the student had any academic problem before. What was missing from consideration is that this student had been here for only a couple of years and his language proficiency in English was still emerging. In fact, during the interview with the student it was clear that he was having trouble processing the questions asked and he needed time and frequent repetitions before he could answer a question. The suggestion was to allow more time for the student to become more proficient in English before he was allowed to proceed with the more demanding components of his academic endeavor. More formal evaluation was discouraged at this point. Psychological treatment was also suggested with someone who has had a similar experience or who was aware of the challenges normally faced by foreign/immigrant students in an academic setting.

Another example was that of a Latino individual already convicted of double murder who was now at the sentencing phase, facing possible capital punishment. He was evaluated in his second language (English) by a group of forensic psychiatrists, including one of a Latino origin. At times, a translator was used to assist in the assessment because the patient's proficiency in English was poor. A final determination was made by this forensic group that the patient engaged in premeditated criminal behavior with no mitigating circumstances and hence capital punishment was being considered by the court. What became clear when evaluating the whole situation was that the patient had a long (and untreated once he immigrated to the United States) history of serious paranoid schizophrenic disorder, from before immigrating to this country, that tended to become easily exacerbated with alcohol abuse. That was not made clear to those responsible for making a determination of culpability (including members of the jury). There were several instances in his personal history of numerous criminal acts, all committed while under the influence, after which the client did not remember what happened. When compensated and less affected by his paranoid condition, the patient presented as a humble, responsible, and agreeable/submissive individual. He was able to keep a job and send money to his family in the country of origin.

When evaluating the assessment performed by the forensic psychiatrists it became evident that it was not clear that the patient understood the questions asked by the psychiatrists or that the psychiatrists understood his answers. The interpreter used was untrained, without the basic knowledge of this patient's unique psychiatric history, and did not have an adequate linguistic (psychiatric concepts) knowledge to be able to translate the patient's verbalization in this regard. The interpretation was fraught with the kinds of errors delineated in Chapter 6 on the use of interpreters. When all these issues were made evident to the judge, the patient was given a life sentence and with a strong recommendation that psychiatric intervention be initiated while incarcerated.

Linguistic Challenges in the Assessment Process

There are various linguistic complications that are normally and inherently present in the assessment of the linguistically diverse individual, like in the cases referred to earlier. These complications are more or less relevant depending on the nature and goal of the assessment. If the assessment seeks to assess an individual's level of cognitive function or ability for learning in the school context, language involvement becomes critical. Although language skills and verbal abilities are closely involved in most aspects of intellectual function and school performance, there are specific functions that are more sensitive to language (and culture) than others (Dana, 1993; Figueroa, 1990; Flanagan et al., 2000). Thus, any task that requires the verbalization of factual information, the ability to make judgments about verbally presented situations, the ability to process progressively more complex verbally presented information, reading comprehension, listening comprehension, vocabulary skills, and writing are all affected by language functioning. It leaves the examiner with an enormous challenge as to how best to assess the cognitive and academic skills of the bilingual individuals who may have different levels of linguistic proficiencies in his or her languages. Failure to ascertain how cultural differences, culturally based behavior, and degree of linguistic proficiency interact with cognitive functioning has resulted in bilingual and culturally diverse individuals to be mislabeled or, in the case of psychiatric condition, misdiagnosed (Javier, 1995; Marcos et al., 1973; Flanagan et al., 2000). For instance, Marcos and associates' bilingual subjects were evaluated as sicker when evaluated in their second and less proficient language. In his analysis, Marcos and associates described a number of linguistic and paralinguistic factors that affected these patients' ability to communicate adequately and for the psychiatrists to be able to appreciate how these patients' responses to their questions were influenced by their unique linguistic difficulties. The research by Marcos and his associates focused on a group of psychiatric patients, representative of the kinds of patients normally seen at that hospital. Their linguistic proficiency in the second language (English) was poor.

Given the description of the bilingual process discussed in previous chapters, it is clear that any assessment of the bilinguals' specific and general cognitive functioning will have to consider the individuals' level of linguistic proficiency as well as the level of synchronicity with the culture of reference (Dana, 1993). We demonstrated in previous chapters how bilingual individuals differ in their linguistic abilities and how information is processed linguistically depending on how the individual learned his or her languages and the level of linguistic proficiency the individual has. When the individual is deficient in the second language and has maintained a subordinate linguistic organization, his or her ability to respond accurately to test questions in a second language will be greatly compromised. We also indicated that we have to show great care even when evaluating a proficient bilingual with a coordinate linguistic organization, since there are cognitive processes that can remain language-specific in terms of its accessibility.

Validity of the Assessment Instruments

Knowing that assessment instruments are developed by a particular society to assess its population with regard to specific dimensions, there is an implicit assumption that the derived scores provide an accurate, valid, and objective appraisal of the individuals' functioning within the cultural and linguistic context in which he or she lives. In the case of academic assessment, it is assumed that it provides a good description of skills and deficiencies that can predict academic achievement and future school success. It is this assumption that is guiding our society's obsession with the development and proliferation of various tests (such as the Wechsler Intelligence scales for children and adults, Woodcock Johnson, Stanford Binet, SAT, GRE, Licensing Exams), including vocational tests and tests to predict marital satisfaction.

Serious challenges have been raised against this assumption, however, from various fronts (Dana, 1993; Helms, 2003; Figueroa, 1990; Flanagan et al., 2000). One of these arguments is that the fact that there are persistent differences in mean IQs of different cultural groups suggests that the test is inherently biased against the groups not included in the standardization of the instrument. Proof of this argument for Helms (2003) is the persistent findings of 200 points lower in SAT-I and one standard deviation lower in intelligence tests for Blacks, as compared to Whites. Following her theory of identity, she found that this effect is particularly pronounced among Blacks who scored high in the identity dimension as African American. According to her, just thinking about being Black affects test scores. In explaining her findings further in the context of her identity theory, she indicated that the Black individual goes through four basic dimensions in his or her identity development:

1. *Conformity* (or stage where identification with the dominant society is strong and operates as if race does not have any bearing)
2. *Dissonance* (or stage of major confusion in which the individual does not feel comfortable with either group)

3. *Immersion* (or stage of great hypersensitivity to race issue, refusing to engage in any activity that is not exclusively Black)
4. *Internalization* (or stage characterized by positive commitment to own racial group)

Racial identity scores significantly predicted test scores for those high in conformity and immersion. When the racial identity scores were removed from the equation, the scores were 313 points higher than those currently found for Blacks. That is, Black scores were 113 points higher than for the White population when they did not think about their racial identity.

Helms emphasized the pernicious and insidious effect of stereotyping in our society in which a group is expected to do worse than another based upon skin colors (2003), cultural, and linguistic backgrounds. Similar analysis was offered by Dana (1993). Such stereotyping, once internalized in the children, functions as a debilitating parasite in the children's mind, setting the stage for the tremendous struggle between the belief of the socially prescribed view of themselves as incapable of performing well and a more positive view of themselves.

According to Flanagan et al., (2000), the fact that a group does systematically poorer than another group in intelligence tests does not make the test invalid. The test is, in fact, doing what it is designed to do, that is, to asses differences between groups. Indeed, according to these authors, the basis verbal-performance factor structure in Wechsler Scales has been, for the most part, reliably replicated in many diverse cultural groups and so the Gc-Gc structure of intelligence; which was found to be invariant across different cultural and racial groups (Flanagan et al., 2000). They reaffirmed Neisser and associates' finding (Neisser et al., 1996) that the IQ derived from the intelligence batteries, as a valid and reliable operationalization of g, is still considered the single best predictor of academic success in the US public school system. That is the case because it reflects the extent to which the individual has been able to assimilate the cultural and linguistic demands, reflected in the test instrument, to succeed in the school system and the society from which the norms were derived. However, these tests may not be able to accurately assess the true nature of the bilingual individual's intellectual capacity in the context of the individual's different linguistic and cultural history, when compared with the mainstream norms.

They proposed a broader approach to assessment that is hypothesis-driven and based on a more ecosystemic framework and interdisciplinary approach in order to obtain data that are less susceptible to cultural discrimination effects and linguistic variations from the mainstream. This cannot be accomplished by simply linguistically adopting or translating a test. This is the case because the underlying assumptions guiding the original test are still operative and hence cannot provide an accurate method for bilingual assessment (Figueroa, 1990; Flanagan et al., 2000). According to these authors, under the best of circumstances, the most valid instrument for a bilingual assessment is one that has been developed and normed in the country where the evaluation is being conducted. For instance, for evaluation in the United States, the test should be developed and normed on US bilingual children, with full consideration of the many possible variant proficiencies in the home language and in English, including the various dialects (Figueroa, 1990; Flanagan et al., 2000). This is truly a time-consuming and very expensive proposition and hence it is not surprising that such a test does not exist today.

And it is in this context that these authors proposed "the selective Wechsler-based Gf-Gc cross-battery approach as a theoretically based method geared at increasing the validity of the assessment of the linguistically/culturally diverse individuals. This method is based on the fact that most intelligence tests, particularly the Wechsler scales, are culturally loaded and that they require language proficiency on the part of both the examiner and examinee. Thus, linguistic factors can affect the administration, comprehension, and performance of even those subtests (e.g., performance subtests) that do not require a verbal response. In their analyses, they divided the different subtests depending on the cultural and linguistic demands on the individual. The reader is encouraged to review Table 8.2 in Flanagan et al. (2000) in which there is a detailed and sophisticated categorization of different subtests for different test instruments in terms of whether the specific subtest has high, moderate, or low linguistic demands or is high, moderate, or low in cultural loading. Table 7.1 provides a summary of such an analysis for Woodcock Johnson's and Wechsler's tests only.

As you can see from the summary table, high in linguistic demands and cultural loading were Similarities, Vocabulary, Information, and Comprehension in the Wechsler's test and Listening Comprehension, Oral Comprehension, Verbal Comprehension, and General Information in the Woodcock Johnson-R/III (WJ-R/III). High in linguistic demands but moderate cultural loading were Incomplete Words and Sound Blending in WJ-RIII, Memory for Words in the WJ-R, and Auditory Attention and Decision Speed in the WJ-III. High in linguistic demands but low in cultural loading are Concept Formation and Analysis Synthesis in WJ-R/III and Auditory Working Memory and Pair Cancellation in the WJ-III. Thus, there are different subtests that are more or less loaded with linguistic demands and/or cultural demands, as shown in Table 7.1 and these demands are to be considered in determining how to proceed with an evaluation in a way that provides the best way to assess a bilingual individual. If we are dealing with a subordinate bilingual, those subtests that are high or moderate in linguistic demands and cultural loading are expected to present great difficulty. The more proficient and culturally integrated the bilingual is, the less the difficulty expected to be experienced with the assessment instruments as a function of the linguistic and cultural loading.

It was this kind of analysis that led Flanagan et al. (2000) to propose a selective Gf-Gc cross-battery approach to assessment, referred to earlier, that allows the assessor to select subtests on the basis of the level of linguistic and cultural loading that best fits the specific need of the individual. (Gf refers to general factors or fluid intelligence thought to include inductive and deducting reasoning and assumed to be influenced by biological and neurological factors and incidental learning through interaction with the environment.

TABLE 7.1. Partial listing of linguistic and cultural loadings of test instrument.

Substest	Test instrument	Age
High linguistic demands and cultural loading		
Similarities	Wechsler's	3–74
Vocabulary	Wechsler's	3–74
Information	Wechsler's	3–74
Comprehension	Wechsler's	3–74
Listening Comprehension	WJ-R	4–85+
Oral Comprehension	WJ-III	4–85+
Verbal Comprehension	WJ-III	2–85+
General Information	WJ-III	2–85+
High linguistic demands and moderate cultural loading		
Incomplete Words	WJ-R/III	2–85+
Sound Blending	WJ-R/III	4–85+
Memory for Words	WJ-R	4–85+
Auditory Attention	WJ-III	4–85+
Decision Speed	WJ-III	4–85+
High linguistic demands and low cultural loading		
Concept Formation	WJ-R/III	4–85+
Analysis Synthesis	WJ-R/III	4–85+
Auditory Working Memory	WJ-III	4–85+
Pair Cancellation	WJ-III	4–85+
Moderate linguistic demands and high cultural loading		
Oral Vocabulary	WJ-R	4–85+
Picture Vocabulary	WJ-R	4–85+
Moderate linguistic demands and cultural loading		
Visual-Auditory Learning	WJ-R/III	4–85+
Delayed Recall-Visual Auditory Learning	WJ-R/III	4–85+
Retrieval Fluency	WJ-III	4–85+
Rapid Picture Naming	WJ-III	4–85+
Arithmetic	Wechsler's	3–74
Moderate linguistic demands and low cultural loading		
Digit Span	WAIS-R	16–74
	WISC-III	6–16
Low linguistic demands and moderate cultural loading		
Object Assembly	Wechsler's	3–74
Picture Recognition	WJ-R/III	4–85+
Visual Closure	WJ-R	2–85+
Low linguistic demands and cultural loading		
Geometric Design	WPPSI-R	3–74

Gc or crystallized intelligence is assumed to consist primarily of abilities that reflect the influences of acculturation, e.g., verbal and conceptual knowledge.) A similar argument was advanced by Armour-Thomas and Gopaul-McNicol (1997) who suggested a more comprehensive system of assessment, such as the Bio-Ecological Assessment System or Bio-Cultural Model of Cognitive Functioning that allows for the inclusion of all relevant information about the individual's true cognitive and emotional ability in the assessment process. The importance of this model is that it emphasizes the centrality of considering other sources of information in making the determination about the level of cognitive functioning. Thus, in the case of a newly immigrant child with poor linguistic skills in English, the Flanagan et al.'s model calls for the tester to avoid those tests that are too loaded in linguistic and cultural demands. For Armour-Thomas and Gopauld-McNicol's model, other sources of information, including a look at how the immigrant child functioned in the country of origin, becomes an essential component of the process and determines its final outcome. The emphasis of both models is on finding areas of strength in the child's overall performance rather than on finding exclusive areas of deficiencies. According to these authors, linguistically and culturally diverse children are more likely to be judged as having learning disability and other cognitive deficiencies and behavioral problems when the assessment instruments utilized are linguistically and culturally inappropriate or the instrument utilized is unable to assess other competences that may be more relevant to the individuals by virtue of their specific reality (Armour-Thomas & Gopaul-McNicol, 1997; Flanagan et al., 2000).

Factors to be Considered in Assessing a Bilingual Individual

What we are saying is that when assessing a bilingual individual, the evaluator should consider a basic set of data including, among other things, degree of bilingualism and bilingual proficiency, as well as extent of acculturation and the basic quality of the test instruments. Thus, whenever possible, the set of data derived from the series of questions listed In table 7.2 should be gathered, as a matter of course, when assessing a linguistically diverse individual. These questions can be informally or more formally explored.

Some of these questions have been suggested by a number of investigators (Cuellar, Arnaldo, & Maldonado, 1995; Cooper, 1975; Lambert et al., 1958; Marin et al., 1987; Javier & Marcos, 1989; Perez-Foster, 1996) as important in assessing linguistic and cultural dimensions in individuals from the diverse community. These authors also proposed specific scales/questionnaires to assess these factors more formally. Thus, I encourage the reader to review these authors' works in this regard. I have also included other questions (particularly the developmental and medical questions) because I have found them to be crucial in assessing bilingual children in general and particularly those who normally come from low socioeconomic levels where conditions related to poverty and plumbism may also be operational and may likely impact negatively on their adequate language functioning (CDC, 1991). For instance, an elevated dentin lead level, even without symptoms of plumbism, has been found to affect speech and language processing in first- and second-grade children (Bellinger, Needleman, Bromfield, & Mintz, 1986). A seminal study by Needleman, Schell, Bellinger, Leviton, and Allred (1990) on the long-term effect of low doses of lead in childhood found that impairment in neurobehavioral function was related to lead content in the teeth in children aged 6 and 7. Young people with dentin lead

TABLE 7.2. Important questions to consider when testing bilingual individuals.

Questions regarding level of linguistic proficiency/cultural competencies:

- *At what age did the subject learn the second language?*
- *In what language and cultural context did the subject have the early schooling?*
- *How long has the subject been in the linguistic/cultural context of the language of the evaluation?*
- *What level of proficiency (in reading, writing, speaking, and thinking?) has the subject reached in the second language?*
- *What level of cognitive/scholastic achievement proficiency did the subject reach in the native language?*
- *What language does the subject use for intellectual/school related material?*
- *In what language does the subject dream?*
- *In what language does the subject think?*
- *What language does the subject prefer when upset or dealing with emotions?*
- *What language is used with whom, for what and under what conditions?*
- *What level of professional accomplishment did the subject reach in the country of origin?*

Questions regarding basic medical/developmental history:

- *When did the subject reach the basic developmental milestones (i.e., walking, language)? This is particularly important in children.*
- *Was there any history of trauma, illnesses, etc. that could have affected the subject's cognitive and linguistic development? Is there a history of lead intoxication and other contaminants? Again, this is particularly important in children.*

level of >20 ppm were found to have a higher risk of dropping out of high school and having reading disability, as compared with those with <10 ppm. A high lead level was also found to produce lower vocabulary and grammatical reasoning scores, increased absenteeism, poorer hand–eyes coordination, longer reaction times, and slower finger tapping. These authors concluded from these findings that exposure to lead in childhood is associated with deficits in the central nervous system functioning that persist into adulthood. Thus, we are left with a question as to what should be expected in the case of bilingual children exposed to lead or other similarly damaging toxins. We are currently analyzing the profile of about 100 bilingual children who were exposed to different levels of lead intoxication at different points in their development. These children were administered a number of cognitive and behavioral tests. We will discuss the findings in a future publication. However, there are some preliminary findings that suggest that the more abstract level of language processing tends to be most affected in these children.

According to Macnamara (1967), as discussed in Chapter 3, a proper assessment of bilingualism must address the relative independence of the languages and the different language domains (e.g., semantic, syntax, and phonology). Thus, it should minimally include reading, writing, and speaking. We will consider a bilingual proficient in the second language when he or she has at least an average level of proficiency in basic skills (reading, writing and speaking) in the second language when compared with native speakers of that language and is able to think, dream, and experience emotions of various kinds in the second language. It is more likely that a bilingual individual with this protocol will have a coordinate or compound linguistic organization. By contrast, a deficient bilingual is expected to have poor proficiency in the basic skills in the second language and it is more likely that he or she will rely on the first language to process information and demands in the second language. It is more likely for a bilingual with this type of protocol to have a subordinate linguistic organization.

Cooper (1975) suggests that a self-report method is an effective and reliable method to assess linguistic proficiency and linguistic organization, and hence there is no need to gather additional data in this regard. In fact, he suggested a questionnaire version that he found to be a strong predictor of linguistic proficiency and organization for bilinguals. According to this author, one can assess degrees of bilingual proficiency by asking the subject to rate his or her level of function in a number of basic skills, comparing with his or her functions of these skills in the primary language, as given in Table 7.3.

We have successfully used these types of questionnaires in our studies (Javier & Marcos, 1989; Javier et al., 1993) but we also advise the inclusion of a vocabulary test and a Global Word Naming test in both languages, to ascertain linguistic proficiency. Thus, for children, one would ask the child to provide definitions of words listed in the vocabulary subtest in English and the translated

TABLE 7.3. Questions to consider in assessing levels of bilingualism and linguistic proficiency.

LINGUISTIC QUESTIONNAIRE
SAMPLE QUESTIONS

1. *If your ability to speak in your primary language is 100 %, how do you rate below your ability to speak in the second language?*
100 %____________________50 %____________________0 %

2. *If your ability to understand in your primary language is 100 %, how do you rate below your ability to understand in the second language?*
100 %____________________50 %____________________0 %

3. *If your ability to read in your primary language is 100 %, how do you rate below your ability to read in the second language?*
100 %____________________50 %____________________0 %

4. *If your ability to write in your primary language is 100 %, how do you rate below your ability to write in the second language?*
100 %____________________50 %____________________0 %

5. *If your ability to think in your primary language is 100 %, how do you rate below your ability to think in the second language?*
100 %____________________50 %____________________0 %

6. *What language do you use, at work, at home, with friends, for intimate communication?*
100 %____________________50 %____________________0 %

7. *In what language do you dream?*
100 %____________________50 %____________________0 %

version of the Wechsler's (e.g., WISC, WISC-R, or WISC-IV), Woodcock Johnson, or Kauffman Assessment Battery for Children (K-ABC). For adult subjects, the vocabulary test in the WAIS will serve this function.

It is important to consider, however, that the fact that vocabulary has a high degree of linguistic and cultural loadings raises serious questions as to whether or not we are truly testing for linguistic proficiency in the subject's two linguistic and cultural contexts when using these tests. Unless the two versions utilized have been standardized in the two linguistic and cultural communities of the subjects under consideration, the fact that a translated version (such as a Spanish version) is utilized does not resolve the problem with contaminations, Anglicisms, alterations of word meanings (Dana, 1993). Nevertheless, even if one only looks at the performance in the English vocabulary version, it provides excellent information about the subject's vocabulary knowledge in English, the subject's second language. Vocabulary performance is often used as good predictor of intellectual and school functioning.

Similarly, the use of the Global Word Naming test may provide a good measure of linguistic proficiency because it compares the subject's performance in this test with itself. It asks the subject to tell as many different words as possible within a minute's time. One can then count and compare (*t*-test) the number of different concepts elicited in the two languages as well as the kinds of concepts in terms of imagery, level of abstraction, and referential activity (Bucci, 1997; Bucci & Freedman, 1978).

Selection of Basic Assessment Instruments

Lopez and Nuñez (1987 and also cited by Dana, 1993) found that the scores of WAIS and EIWA (Spanish version) were not comparable and suggested that assessors should use the EIWA, instead of the WAIS or WAIS-R, with language-impaired and minimally educated subjects, since that was the population utilized for its (that of the EIWA) standardization. Similar findings were reported by Gonzalez (2002) in a study that used four test conditions: WAIS condition (or condition that tested a group of coordinate bilinguals with the WAIS scales as developed), a WAIS Spanish version condition (or condition that tested a group of coordinate bilinguals in a Spanish or translated version of the WAIS that preserved its basic structure), an EIWA condition (or condition that tested a group of coordinate bilinguals in Spanish in the way that the scale was developed), and finally, an EIWA English version (or a condition that tested a group of coordinate bilinguals with a translated version of the EIWA in English that preserved the original structure of the EIWA). It was clear that the two tests have different structures and the nature and findings derived from these instruments were not comparable.

According to Dana (1993), similar statements can be made with regard to other translated instruments, such as the Chinese translations of the WISC and the WAIS, where proper standardization was questionable. He suggested that before a decision is made about a specific instrument, the assessor "should be informed of the specific data used for interpretations of cognitive functioning and the normative data used as a basis for these interpretations" (p. 187). He even suggested the need to rely on other sources of information to arrive at a decision about cognitive functioning.

Thus, when dealing with bilinguals with limited English language proficiency (a subordinate bilingual), we need to be aware of the nature of the tests utilized and avoid tests that are too linguistically and culturally loaded, and if used, interpretations should be made with caution. In this context, the Kaufman Assessment Battery for Children (K-ABC) has been found to result in less IQ differences among Hispanic Americans, African Americans, and Anglo Americans than when using the WISC-R (Dana, 1993). The more acculturated and proficient the subject is in the language of the test (English), the less concern there is about the accuracy and validity of the findings. For bilinguals at the coordinate/compound proficient spectrum who are highly acculturated, it is less likely to matter whether the test instruments utilized is linguistically and/or culturally loaded. By contrast, for bilinguals with a subordinate and deficient linguistic organization and with low acculturation, a test like the K-ABC is more appropriate. If the Wechsler and the Woodcock Johnson tests have to be utilized in spite of the concerns raised in this chapter, it will be more appropriate to use the subject's primary language as the language of test.

8
Treatment of the Bilingual Patients

In previous chapters we have described the extent to which language is involved in most aspects of the individual's cognitive development, including memory organization. We have emphasized how experiences are organized linguistically, having a direct effect on the development of the self and memories normally associated with the major developmental milestones. In this chapter, I will further discuss the way the bilingual's languages are intimately connected to the emotional life of the bilingual person and how they emerge in the context of a treatment experience. Most of the information presented here has been derived from direct observations and treatment of bilingual patients. Although we will use a psychoanalytic perspective to illustrate our thesis, any point made here will also apply to any treatment perspective that relies on verbal communication for the purpose of assessment and intervention.

Our concern with identifying emotional factors that may impact on memory accessibility in bilinguals is based on our observation of the additional complications brought about in the treatment of these patients, who, by definition, have more than one linguistic code to process and organize events, perceptions, and experiences in their lives. I have discussed some of these complications in previous publications in which I suggested that the nature and extent of the retrievability of a memory is greatly affected by the quality of the individual's linguistic and psychic organization (Javier, 1989), in addition to the neurolinguistic condition already referred to by Paradis (2003) and discussed in previous chapters. By psychic organization I am referring to the internal (psychological) organization that gives rise to mentation and cognitive and emotional organization influenced by factors not always within the subject's consciousness (Figure 8.1). This internal (psychic) organization includes the individual's self-definition, self and group identities, belief and value systems, worldviews and personality characteristics that guide his or her perception and relation with the world and the self.

Thus, we recognize that by also incorporating analyses of the linguistic processes associated with these aspects of the individual's internal organization, it may be possible to reach a fuller understanding and appreciation of these individuals' true psychological (internal) structure motivating their behavior. In Figure 8.1 the reader may be able to visualize the multiple levels of organization that take place and that result in what we then call the "Bilingual Individual." With regard to the treatment situation, it is our contention that only by incorporating analyses of the linguistic processes in the treatment equation can we obviate the danger of what Judith Welles (1993) called "counterfeit analyses;

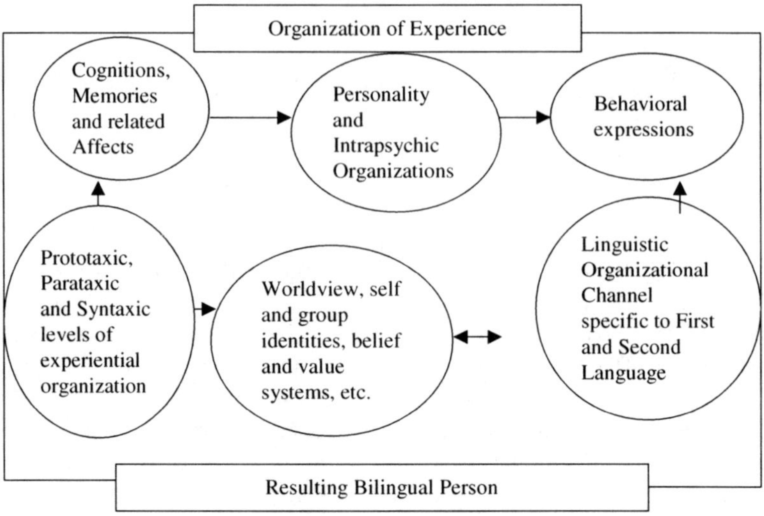

FIGURE 8.1. Personality formation in a bilingual context.

maintaining the illusion of knowing." Counterfeit refers to a situation in which the true nature and content of the communication remain hidden or incomplete due to a linguistic confusion or compromised emotional state that leaves essential aspects of the individual's internal (psychic) structure that is connected to his or her unique relation to his or her languages, inaccessible and hence not part of the treatment situation.

The belief that the quality and nature of the psychological organization could be affected by the linguistic organization of the individual under consideration is based upon empirical data (Javier & Marcos, 1989; Javier et al., 1993) and psychoanalytic observations of patients who showed different qualities of memories depending on the languages utilized to express these memories and whose treatments were characterized by complex displays of linguistic switching as important (traumatic) memories were being discussed (Buxbaum, 1949; Greenson, 1950; Javier, 1995). When the treatment situation's main goal is to help the person regain access to memory contents that are out of the individual's awareness (like in the case of psychoanalytic treatment) then it provides the individual with an opportunity to reconstruct his or her past.

As discussed in an earlier publication (Javier, 1996), in psychological and psychoanalytic thinking, memory reconstruction does not imply the creation of a memory that never occurred, but the reconstruction of a memory, which, though remaining inaccessible due to psychic factors, has influenced the nature of the individual's experience. An essential aspect of psychological/psychoanalytic exploration is the search for "what" the experience is all about, "where" it took place, "who" was involved in the experience, and "when" it occurred. These are the kinds of experience attributes that make it possible to establish the memory of an experience with some degree of certainty (Wagenaar, 1986). Thus, this type of inquiry does not leave much room for repressed "false" memories because it is less likely for these types of memories to withstand the power of psychoanalytic scrutiny.

With regard to psychoanalytic formulation, the emphasis of psychoanalytic scrutiny is on the examination of an individual's character structure, which has been influenced by infantile conflictual memories, and the examination of these memories without concern for the extent to which they maintain any resemblance to objectively proven reality. That is, psychoanalytic exploration is concerned with psychic reality, or a mental set created by persistent unconscious conflictual factors (Arlow, 1985). It is not possible to prove with any degree of certainty the extent to which early memories of past events are accurate with regard to the "who," "when," and "where." According to Cohen (1989) and Wagenaar (1986), only "what" the experience was all about seems to provide a categorical organization of the experience that is likely to be remembered more accurately.

Memory Organization in Bilingual Patients

The following clinical case is meant to provide an example of how the factors discussed above appear in the treatment situation. It refers to a case that was discussed in an early publication (Javier, 1996) and that I decided to present here again because of its richness with regard to the issues of concern. This is a summary of the treatment of a young bilingual individual who spent his first few formative years traveling to various countries as his father was transferred from one diplomatic post to another. At home, there were various languages spoken depending upon whether the immediate family was alone or accompanied by friends and acquaintances or family members who only spoke one of the languages. The patient, having become proficient in a second language, felt comfortable interchanging his languages as the occasion demanded it. He reported not finding much pleasure in things he was doing especially when he felt that he was obliged to do them. This was one of the reasons for seeking treatment and, although he initially requested treatment in the primary language, he started his sessions in his second language, speaking in a precise manner about his pain.

He was a talented young man in the arts and sports and also in his chosen profession. He was frequently admired by his supervisors and colleagues but responded to praise in a mixed manner as he felt that more was going to be demanded of him by those praising him. Although he frequently described what appeared to be intense feelings in reference to these experiences, his voice remained monotone, even when tears started to come down his cheek. There was a quality of detachment in his presentation. There was a sense of depression in him, often finding himself sad and moody as if about to cry without knowing why. This was, in fact, one of the reasons for his seeking treatment. He came to his sessions on time, but it was clear that he did not feel comfortable in the treatment situation. At times, he would even become mute in his treatment, unable to find words to describe his feelings.

Memories from his past were presented factually and devoid of any personal texture, after which he would start to sob. He often verbalized feelings of not being sure where he wanted to live, whether it was better for him to stay in the city, to move to the suburbs or to just leave the country altogether. He described himself as terribly afraid of planes and of the dark, and walked around with a general feeling of catastrophe. What really transpired in this patient's past so as to give him this sense of fragmentation and general feeling that he was not quite where he was supposed to be? To answer that question, it was important to get into a careful reconstruction of this patient's past by a systematic gathering of aspects of his personal history and early memories.

Memory reconstruction and its related phenomenon, repression, constitute the cornerstone of psychoanalytic conceptualization and practice (Freud, 1914). In Freudian conceptualization, ordinary perceptions, thoughts, motivations, fantasies, wishes, dreams, and memories of events as well as the individual's relationship with himself or herself and others are influenced by the vicissitudes of unconscious fantasies and conflictual demands made by Id–Ego–Superego processes on the mental life of the individual (Brenner, 1979; Bucci, 1985; Freud, 1940). As stated before, this is what has been referred to as psychic reality, or the mental set created by persistent unconscious fantasies (Arlow, 1985; Freud, 1896, 1905, 1940).

It is against this mental set that "the data of perception are perceived, registered, interpreted, remembered, and responded to" (Arlow, 1985, p. 526). In this context, neurotic processes, and transference manifestation for that matter, can be said to represent how the "individual misperceives, misinterprets, and misresponds to the data of perception in terms of the mental set created by persistent unconscious fantasies." They represent the work of repressed memories that find expression through these means.

Freud (1940) recognized that because of the quality and nature of mental representation and the possibility for distortion due to the work of the unconscious, it is difficult and even impossible to accurately and objectively ascertain, with any degree of certainty, a mental representation's real components. Thus, his reliance on inferences and interpolations constituted the basic elements of his psychoanalytic method, the technique that provides the best opportunity to reach inaccessible (repressed) memories of events.

In the case of our patient, it was clear by the nature of his complaints, the symptomatic transformations (phobias) reported, as well as his linguistic history that a sense of the nature of his psychic reality could only be obtained in the context of his multilinguistic reality. It was also clear that although the patient only remembered experiencing these types of symptoms for the last few years, the quality of the symptoms could not be explained unless they were seen in the context of his much earlier experiences. For instance, he was able to speak about a number of apparently important experiences while in other countries: his piano and art lessons, the friends he made along the way, his language teacher and the many hours he spent alone in his room, the time his father never made it to his piano recital, and his relief when he finally saw his mother in the audience. The patient was surprised that he would feel irritable after expressing these types of experiences and his behavior following these sessions would become characterized by silence and a reluctance to get into any thing "heavy." He would then apologize. Similar reactions were observed in another bilingual patient discussed in a previous paper (Javier, 1995).

The patient was unable to bring any understanding to his feeling of irritability, other than feeling that these were very personal moments that he had not discussed with anybody. Nevertheless, he was very respectful with me and was very eager to please me by trying to give whatever association he thought I wanted from him. And even after these types of sessions, he would frequently verbalize his satisfaction with the treatment. Were we in the midst of a resistance, or was the patient attempting to communicate another important aspect of his experience in which compliance was the safest way of being? Being satisfied in this context was a way of saying that it was a familiar position, although the nature of this was not totally within his awareness.

Nature of Memory Inaccessibility in a Bilingual Context

The careful examination of the bilingual individuals' verbalization provides us with a wonderful opportunity to examine important concepts in psychology and mental health pertaining to memory and accessibility of information. Can we assume that an experience is being repressed or is out of cognitive awareness when we are dealing with an individual who possesses two different linguistic codes to organize and process his or her experience?

Jones' (1993) excellent discussion on the evolution of the concept of depression can be instrumental in helping us understand the different levels of repression (or inaccessibility of experience) in our patient. In this article, she examined the evolution of the concept of repression from the more normal process to repression proper, or what Bucci (1985) refers to as "complete and persistent inaccessibility of representations, resulting from their association with anxiety and other painful affect" (p. 590). Jones eloquently discussed various kinds of repression possible, each with various implications for psychoanalytic conceptualization. Of those discussed, only four seem to be relevant for our discussion:

1. Preverbal infantile repression
2. Postverbal infantile repression
3. State dependent repression, and
4. Repression proper (which can occur as part of an automatized suppression mechanism or as part of a conditioned repression mechanism).

Preverbal infantile repression refers to those experiences, feelings, and wishes that were encoded in a nonverbal form (or perceptual–sensory channel) and are thus not accessible to verbal, that is, conscious recall. According to Jones (1993):

The nonverbal memory whose reemergence is stimulated by the evolution of the transference finds its way to verbal representation in a highly disguised form, similar to dream representation. The complex feelings surrounding the traumatic event are then able to be worked through verbally in the analysis. (p. 86)

Postverbal infantile repression, on the other hand, refers to a condition in which "certain experiences, affects, or drive derivatives are nevertheless experienced and encoded in nonverbal form" (Jones, 1993, p. 86), although development of language has already taken place. As is the case with preverbal infantile depression, memories associated with this state of depression can become available through the transference, which then becomes the vehicle for verbal expression of the experience. Initially, however, these two types of depressions are experienced in a more somatic–sensory form. In a more general way we can define 'transference' as a process by which an individual is able to project/connect to someone in the present feelings/memories from the past that are not within the conscious awareness of this individual. By so doing, these feelings/memories can become more accessible to this individual's conscious awareness in the present.

In the case of a state-dependent repression "an experience, feeling, or wish occurring in the past may be inaccessible to consciousness because the individual was in an altered state of consciousness at the time of its occurrence" (p. 87), so that it may be possible for the individual to retrieve the specific memory if that altered state of consciousness is recreated. With regard to the bilingual process, we can also say that a kind of altered state of consciousness is developed when a patient processes aspects of a traumatic experience in a specific linguistic mode (one of the languages), which then remain inaccessible to consciousness until he or she can return to that state of linguistic mind.

Unlike the previous repressions, the crucial element of repression proper has to do with a condition in which feelings, wishes, and fantasies that were at one point unquestionably in conscious awareness and accessible to verbal representation are now inaccessible "due to the mobilization of guilt, shame, or disgust" (Jones, 1993, p. 88). Thus, the crucial differences among all these levels of inaccessibility of the experience is that only the latter constitutes a true repression, as usually defined in the psychoanalytic literature. The others may be explained through mechanisms related to linguistic maturational processes and linguistic inaccessibility.

We find that the distinctions of the different kinds of depressive experience made by Jones as very useful in helping us make sense of our patient's experience. We can see, for instance, that the fact that our patient registered irritability and then was unable to communicate verbally suggests that perhaps we were dealing with repressed memories of a preverbal infantile nature, a state-dependent condition or at the very least with an experience that has remained organized at the "perceptual channel" of the kinds referred to as postverbal infantile repression. If that is the case, how are we to help the patient have access to the information? We suspect that the success of the analysis of this patient would depend not so much on the language utilized (he is proficient in his languages) but on the extent to which the patient is able to return to that state of psychic representation associated with the conflictual experience under discussion. What we discovered with this patient was that he responded very strongly when the primary language was introduced inadvertently (or was it?) by me at the beginning of a session, following a number of sessions in which the patient appeared rather detached while talking about his father. During these sessions his father was described as removed and uninvolved with the family affairs but he also remembered feeling close to him while he was small. Details of these experiences, however, were vague and sketchy. His description of his mother, on the other hand, was much more vivid and present: He remembered her driving him to school, her involvement in his piano and art lessons, the food she prepared, her responses to his illnesses, etc. Again, the feeling of irritability would emerge after these sessions.

After the primary language was introduced (when I asked the patient to "come in" in his primary language), a much more complex sense of the father emerged. He remembered his father as always in social meetings, hosting parties for friends and colleagues when he was not at home. When at home, on the other hand, the patient remembered him as always retreating to his study room alone to unwind, leaving the patient with an experience of a father as distant and unavailable. Nevertheless, he still harbored a great deal of admiration for him. He felt that, in many ways, he resembled his father in many of the things he did. He described himself as a thinker, like his father, and it was clear that he was favored over his sister. He remembered with great longing a time at the beach playing ball when he was 5 years old. The father had taken two weeks off before being transferred to another foreign diplomatic post and went away with the family to the beach. Although the patient had been at the beach several times with his mother, he remembered this time the most: the salty and warm water, the white sand, the kiosk by the water where he ran with his father to buy a vanilla ice cream. It was a vivid description of a time when his relationship with his dad was the most rewarding, after which the patient felt a sense of warmth toward his father.

Following these verbalizations, the patient again reported feeling in a bad mood at work and at home. He felt angry at his father and depressed. Angry because these types of experiences were few and far apart, and because he remembered always waiting for his father to come home from work and finally falling asleep without seeing him. After only a few sessions speaking in the primary language, the patient then decided to return to the second language, abruptly stating that he did not feel comfortable speaking in the first language, "that it was not appropriate." I suspected that the patient was getting in touch with his rage toward his father and desperately needed to gain some distance, which the second language provided, in order to preserve his image of the father.

What is so interesting in the treatment of this patient is that he became petrified and overwhelmed with emotion when he heard his first language being spoken by the therapist. The patient had been able to talk in detail about a number of important memories; but there was a sense that something was missing from the memories, especially with regard to his father. His descriptions were stale as if missing texture and warmth. After allowing memories of the father that developed in the context of the first language to emerge, his verbalization in the second language also became characterized with a kind of richness and texture not felt until then. This phenomenon was also experimentally demonstrated by Javier and colleagues (1993) in a psycholinguistic study discussed earlier in this book. For this patient, as with previous ones, we could see the interplay of language and the psychic state and hence the importance of submitting both to the same kind of analytic inquiry.

The extent to which the patient was able to speak about his conflictual experience with his father but not be fully aware of the range of his affective responses suggests that repression in the form of isolation of affects can be said to have taken place. But, to the extent to which the shifting of the language allowed for a more full expression of the experience, it suggests that a "state-dependent repression" had taken place. However, the fact that the patient seemed to lack the linguistic symbolism to relate his early experience with his dad in a vivid manner in his second language but was able to do so in the first language suggests that a combination of state-dependent repression and preverbal infantile repression, or perhaps postverbal infantile repression, may have been in operation.

An inaccessibility of an experience does not in itself reflect the work of repression proper since such inaccessibility could be linguistically based, although for some material repression proper may also be involved. From that perspective, it can be said that in the case of some experiences, the richness of the memories may emerge more clearly when the language closer to the experience is in operation than when it is not. For other experiences, it may be possible for the assumed "repressed memories" to find ways of expression in the context of the analysis even in the language originally most distant from the experience. In a case of a bilingual who is deficient in a second language, however, this may be much more complicated as repression of the experience may be further exacerbated in the second language (Marcos & Alpert, 1976), because the individual may not possess adequate linguistic symbols to communicate the experience.

Technical Considerations

In view of the complexity of the linguistic and psychic process, it would be difficult to provide specific technical comments as to the best way to proceed with the treatment of bilingual patients. I have tried to advance the proposition that the treatment of individuals who have more than one language to organize and communicate their experiences cannot be understood adequately outside the context of the individual's personal psychology, or the nature of his or her psychic reality. What is important is to reach with the patient a state of "transforming dialogue" (Wolff, 1988) and that Freedman (1983) further describes in his article "On psychoanalytic listening." In this article he suggests that all listening involves a sequence of rhythmic alternation of two phases: receiving and restructuring. During the phase of receiving there is "... an openness to the intent of the other ... a tolerance for multiple alternatives ... an emphasis on subjectivity, that is, a suspension of the need to objectify or symbolize" (p. 409). During the phase of restructuring, on the other hand, there is "... a narrowing of attention, a reduction of the possibilities aiming toward consolidation and synthesis, and emphasis of objectification and symbolic representation" (p. 409). For a proper receiving phase to occur, the therapist should be able to form clear images in his or her mind (not concepts) from the patient's verbalization, including the affective components of the experience(s) verbalized by the patient. Only in this manner, development of true empathy for the patient's dilemma may be possible. The restructuring process should only begin when the image is fixed securely and vividly in the therapist's mind. In this regard, if the therapist is successful in establishing this kind of dialogue with bilingual patients, and the linguistic behavior is seen in the context of the linguistic characteristics and the nature of the patient's psychic condition, it is likely that the treatment will progress as expected and the danger of a counterfeit treatment would be avoided.

These considerations are applicable to any treatment situation that relies on verbal communication to foster change in the patient's condition. In this context, cognitive behavioral or rational emotive therapy should also pay particular attention to these considerations because their interventions could be rendered ineffective by the nature and quality of the linguistic organization of the patient. So, attempting to eradicate belief systems that were developed during the early developmental years and that are closely associated with the patient's first language could be rendered less effective if done in the patient's second language. This is particularly the case for a patient who is prone to intellectualization and may use the second language production as a distancing device to ward off the affective components associated with development of these beliefs. On the other hand, if the patient is fraught with too much anxiety related to these beliefs, dealing with the issue in the second language initially may produce the necessary therapeutic environment to address the issue under less disruptive conditions for the patient. Eventually, addressing these beliefs in the person's first language, if possible, could provide the most complete intervention.

Those involved in treatment of family or group therapy may find it quite challenging to ensure that the communication between and among bilingual participants are, indeed, at the same level in terms of the intended contents of the communication and the range of emotions normally associated with these contents. Thus, making a brief language assessment of the participants' linguistic history and proficiency, as suggested earlier in Chapter 7, could provide the professional with the best possibility to place these communications in the context of the participants' unique personal and linguistic history. For each participant to then recognize their unique bilingual quality of communication and the unique bilingual quality of the other participants will allow the therapist to address the multiple ways in which communication of needs could be distorted as a function of personal, family, or group dynamics, the participants' unique linguistic organization and proficiency, and/or the combination of all these.

Conclusion

Memory reconstruction and its related phenomenon, repression, constitute the cornerstone of psychoanalytic and psychodynamic conceptualization and practice. Indeed, it is the role of analytic/psychodynamic treatment to help the patient reclaim past memories and thus establish a different and more cohesive and integrated view or personal narrative of the past with the present (Arlow, 1985; Freeman, 1985; Wallerstein, 1985). This suggests that the working through of repressed painful memories can result in a different reorganization of the internal (psychic) structure under more conscious control. Thus, the analysis of processes such as superego functions and the vicissitude of the Id and its derivatives, the analysis of transference and countertransference, and dream interpretations all serve important roles in working through unconscious material. In the case of bilinguals, an analytic/dynamic treatment that does not also include the role of his or her language in the quality of the internal makeup can only lead to a counterfeit transaction in which both the treating professional and the patient can only maintain the "illusion of knowing" the true content of the patient's communication.

As we suggested earlier, it is important, when dealing with bilingual patients, to always make sure to evaluate in some way the level of language proficiency of the patient in both languages, the history of the linguistic development of both languages in the context of the psychological development history, language-specific experiences, and the like. Otherwise, the therapist may have difficulty recognizing when the problem exhibited by the patient regarding accessibility of specific memories may be partly due to his bilingual experience. The importance of language assessment was also stressed by Perez-Foster (1996) as an essential part of any treatment intervention with bilinguals. She provides the reader with an excellent and concrete way to incorporate an assessment of the patient's personal experience in the context of his or her linguistic history. It can be a powerful tool to reach important memories in the patient's personal history if it is used in the dynamic way intended by the author.

9
Future of Bilingualism: What Should be Our Response?

In previous chapters our attention focused, among other things, on the description of bilingualism, characteristics of the bilingual brain, issues of linguistic organization, role of language in cognitive and emotional processes, issues on assessing the bilingual individual and treatment issues. In the context of these discussions, we presented different arguments from the literature delineating the importance of looking at the bilingual experience and some of the obstacles in considering the benefit of bilingualism in our society. The argument that bilingualism results in cognitive difficulty, split identity, cultural dislocation, and poor self-image at the individual level, and in regional and national disunity and intergroup conflict at the society level, has not found much support in the literature (Baker, 1993). Nevertheless, such an argument continues to influence many decisions made about the appropriateness/benefits of teaching a second language, of learning in a second language, the importance of retaining one's primary language, and the importance of bilingual education. At the heart of the argument is a strong but unprocessed and perhaps unconscious anxiety/belief that the only way to retain a national identity is through total assimilation of cultures and languages. Inherent in the argument is also a strong anti-immigrant sentiment. Thus, the greatest threat to bilingualism is the prevailing negative attitude and personal/society anxiety that individuals in the society with decision-making power (such as politicians) still maintain against linguistically diverse and immigrant individuals. This basic attitude (personal prejudice) has influenced the different solutions to questions related to bilingualism, the bilingual individual, and the societal needs and has created an inability to provide more comprehensive solutions to the problem.

Traditional Response

There are a number of factors that have contributed to creating a certain urgency in those involved in human services to come up with a better solution to the linguistic needs of linguistically diverse immigrants than the one maintained up to now. As indicated in Chapter 1, the world has become more linguistically diverse as a result of increased immigration, globalization, and proliferation of technology that make communication between and among different linguistic communities more possible. This increase in linguistically diverse populations has permeated all aspects of our society, but particularly our schools, hospitals, legal systems, etc. In fact, there are believed to be 5.5 to 6.3 million students with limited English proficiency in the United States (Flanagan et al., 2000), and this figure is expected to increase even more, particularly among the Spanish speaking that already comprise more than 12.5% of the total population (U.S. Census, 2002). Specifically in New York, only 52% or almost 6 million New Yorkers surveyed are native speakers of English and 48% are not. The overwhelming majority of those 48% (or 51%) speak Spanish at home, followed by Chinese (13%), Russian (8%), French (4%), Korean, and Italian (3% each). Bialystok and Cummings (2000) reporting data from a 1987 survey of seven European countries by the Center for Educational Research and Innovation (CERI) of the Organization for Economic Co-operation and Development (OECD) describe the population shift in the educational population in these countries. The average foreign enrolment ranged from 4.8 % in the Netherlands to 18% in Switzerland, 38% in Luxembourg, 13.5% in Belgium, 10.1% in France, 11.9% in Germany and 8.7% in Sweden. According to these authors, the magnitude of this population shift can be seen in the net loss of 1.1 million German children and a gain of 400,000 foreign children between the years 1974/1975 and 1981/1982. These authors also reported a similar population shift in California where the proportion of the limited-English-proficient students rose by 14% between 1988 and 1989.

The resulting impact on curriculum development, teacher preparation, nature and quality of classroom material is unparalleled and challenges the traditional way of looking at education and learning and the way our teachers are prepared. We are no longer dealing with a monolithic population of individuals with similar needs and characteristics, but now diverse linguistic and cultural-based learning styles and ways of processing cognitive information and affect are integral parts of the educational demands and intimately involved in the evaluation and treatment of these individuals.

Two major thrusts have guided the different programs utilized to address the needs of linguistically diverse immigrants. One is guided by the belief that the quick and immediate assimilation of the linguistically diverse immigrant groups will help maximize and adjust faster and better into the host society. Thus, all instructions should be in English from the very beginning and students will be expected to command the second language within a specific time. The other is guided by the belief that such assimilation should occur gradually and by considering the utilization of the native language as a transitional tool to accomplish the linguistic assimilation. The former is embodied in the "English only" movement and the latter in the "English plus" movement (Baker, 1993).

Those in support of "English only" argument raised a questionable (and a rather political) argument that minority language is often connected with poverty, underachievement in school, minimal social and vocational mobility, and lack of integration with the majority (Baker, 1993). Thus, a bilingual education is considered more harmful than helpful in facilitating the adequate adjustment into the host society (Imoff, 1990). Those in support of a more flexible approach are concerned with developing a less traumatic condition where learning could take place in the context of other psychological developments, such as self-esteem, positive attitude to schooling, self-identity, and sense of well-being and cohesiveness. In fact, according to Baker (1993), a strong bilingual education can lead to higher achievement across the curriculum for the minority language children, and can foster self-esteem, self-identity, and positive attitude toward schooling. Being able to maintain the home language and culture fosters feelings of well-being and cohesiveness.

The fact that in the "English only" movement having a minority language is seen as a problem and liability rather than an asset, reveals a fundamental bias and belief system against minority languages, minority cultures, and the immigrants. Such a negative belief is likely to contaminate the learning experience of the language minority individuals in that there will be less opportunity to allow educational programs that consider their specific linguistic and educational needs. As we said earlier, language minority individuals have different levels of linguistic proficiency and linguistic dominance and hence educational intervention should keep these qualities into consideration.

Another consequence inherent in the "English only" movement is reflected in the manner with which our society has attempted to address the issue of the diverse linguistic community referred to earlier. That is, to marginalize those who, for one reason or another, decide to retain close contacts with their languages and cultures. It is in this way that the various marginal groups were formed in many European cities and cities in the United States (Grosjean, 1989; Miller, 1991). Although rapidly changing with the economic power amassed by these linguistic groups, the Hispanic/Latino and Asian individuals have been identified as part of these marginal and stigmatized groups in the United States. Other groups include the Polish, Italian, Greek, Hasidic Jew, Haitian, and now the Russian who have also formed enclaves in various parts of metropolitan areas where their customs, cultures, religions, and languages are preserved in various degrees.

There is No Easy Solution to the Bilingual Dilemma

All specifically human psychological processes (higher mental processes) are mediated by psychological tools, including languages, signs, and symbols (Kaspov & Haywood, 1998; Vygotsky, 1962). Vygotsky's view of the centrality of language in human condition is summarized by Karpov and Haywood (1998):

> Language enables children to provide for auxiliary tools in the solution of difficult tasks, to overcome impulsive action, to plan a solution to a problem prior to its execution and to master their own behavior. (p. 28)

Thus, language serves a fundamental role in mediating cognitive and metacognitive processes. As demonstrated in previous chapters, bilingualism presents an additional challenge to the bilingual individuals themselves and those involved in teaching, evaluating, and treating bilingual individuals. What language is used for mediation of the individual's psychological processes will be a function of what language was used for the development of the specific processes under consideration, the nature of the bilingual organization, and the level of linguistic proficiency. For instance, if one asks a bilingual individual what is the preferred language for a specific cognitive process (e.g., thinking, dreaming, mental computation), the answer to that question will depend on the language involved in the development of these processes. Vaid and Menon (2000) found in this regard, that the language of instruction was the strongest predictor of language preference for mental arithmetic (procedural knowledge), followed by length of residence in the United States, onset of bilingualism, and relative language dominance. Language of instruction, length of residence, and relative language dominance also predicted the language preference for thinking to oneself and dreaming but in different ways. In the case of thinking, the best predictor was length of residence, followed by the language of elementary instruction, followed by language proficiency. In the case of dreaming, the best predictor was language dominance, followed by length of residence, followed by language of elementary instruction.

Thus, a decision of what language to use to address the different needs of the bilingual individuals will depend on the mental activities under consideration in addition to the specific characteristics of the bilingual individuals. That is, not all bilinguals are the same with regard to needs and hence any programmatic intervention should consider these characteristics if it is going to be successful. In this context, an educational system that forces the linguistic minority individuals into an immersion bilingual program or transitional bilingual program or a program that includes a bilingual unit within a mainstream school system will only be successful for those bilinguals for whom their linguistic history and prior educational experience will make it possible to benefit from these types of programs. An immersion program for linguistic minority individuals with deficient linguistic knowledge in the second language is likely to be successful for those individuals with good linguistic knowledge in the native language and good attitude toward bilingualism. An example of this level of success is found in Canada (Baker, 1993). It is also found in my own observations and anecdotal stories of some individuals in bilingual programs in New York City whose level of preparation in the native language was superior to that of those in the bilingual program and who decided to completely immerse themselves in English to the dismay and criticism of their colleagues. For some of these individuals, learning the second language was experienced as giving up on a society from which they felt politically and economically alienated. Those who ventured into an immersion program saw learning the language as an important opportunity to take advantage and partake of the educational, political, and economic possibilities. They saw it as an opportunity to expand on their ability to process information in different linguistic modes. This is in keeping with the findings reported by Bialystok and Cummins (2000) that there is a strong relationship between literacy and between first and second languages. Bilingual children were found to experience more varied possibilities for language processing, which may also result in cognitive and academic advantages.

It is not surprising, then, that Hispanic students with several years of school in Latin America were reported to have better academic prospects than Hispanic students born in the United States who, in turn, performed as poorly as Black students (Cummins, 1989, 1991). This suggests that the linguistic mismatches should not be the only aspect of concern when dealing with the linguistic minority; cultural mismatches should also be considered (Armour-Thomas & Gopaul- McNicol, 1997; Flanagan et al., 2000). It also supports Cummins' contention (1986, also cited by Baker, 1993) that when language minority students are instructed through the minority language for all or part of the school day, they perform as well in English academic skills as comparable students instructed totally through English (Baker, 1993). According to Cummins (2000), there is no evidence that bilingual instruction impedes children's acquisition of literacy in the majority language. Cummins also suggested that the transfer of proficiency acquired through minority language learning will occur given adequate exposure and motivation to learn the language. Finally, he suggested that the quality of context in which the educational experience takes place is crucial. That is, community, school characteristics, power, and status relationships all need to be considered in the development of a proper bilingual education program (cited by Baker, 1993).

Thus, the most adequate solution to the bilingual dilemma requires a flexible structure where the areas delineated in Table 9.1 are considered (Baker, 1993; Bialystok, 2000):

The need for a more flexible structure in dealing with the bilingual individual has been proposed by a number of scholars over the years based on solid research data (Bialystok & Cummins, 2000). Nevertheless, our society continues to flounder for an answer to the bilingual question because, as we said earlier, a flexible approach to bilingualism calls for a change in the traditional paradigm. It requires a realignment of priority and basic attitude toward the minority languages. It requires a reallocation of resources to allow for better preparation of teachers, flexible curriculum designs, more diverse instructional material, more differentiated conception of competencies of bilingual individuals, more culturally sensitive school environment, etc. It requires supporting/encouraging more systematic research on learning in two languages, learning in a second language, curriculum development, learning style, etc. Finally, it requires giving up on the fear of disunity assumed to result from allowing members in the society to maintain more than one language.

It is instructive to recognize the important role that this fear of disunity or total disintegration of our society played in the Civil War in that it propelled the Union forces to prevail against the Confederate forces that were looking

TABLE 9.1. Different factors to be considered when developing an educational intervention.

Intervention Components
a) Individual characteristics
• The individual's level of linguistic proficiency
• Academic level/competencies reached in the primary language
• Age of the second language acquisition
• Level of linguistic dominance
• Length of residence in the second language
b) *Task characteristics*
• Nature of tasks/mental activity under consideration
• Language involved in the acquisition of the skills under consideration
c) *Learning environment*
• Nature of the learning environment
• Preparation of the teachers
• Quality of instructional material
• Adequacy of the curriculum and instruction
• Resources available
d) *Society characteristics*
• Society attitude toward the minority language

for less centralized government. The United States was a still a young country then and was still struggling to establish its identity. Thus, having a common language was of the utmost importance, as was having a common constitution of government. We can see a similar process in place in the way the Catholic Church required, before the Vatican II Council, that all rituals be performed in Latin at all the churches around the world and thus foster a universal unity at that level. Allowing the churches to use vernacular languages for ritual made it possible for the participants to become more involved in and understand the rituals. Latin still remained the language of the Church, as we were able to witness in the recent funeral of Pope John Paul II.

The flexible approach suggested earlier requires allocation of funds and commitment that many of our elected and governmental officials may not be prepared to do. But the consequence for our society is to still remain unprepared to address the challenges associated with an increasingly linguistically and culturally diverse society. We discussed in the introductory chapter the most recent danger in the Iraq War and the war on terrorism of not having linguistically sophisticated personnel in the military/intelligence units to allow for better communication of information among those involved in these conflicts. The business community is aware of the buying power that some immigrant groups (e.g., Latino, Asian, Russian) have and hence is now paying more attention to these groups in terms of linguistically/culturally sensitive advertisements.

There Are Signs of Hope

Unlike the prevalent attitudes previously maintained by individuals with different linguistic histories, bilingual groups are now demanding more understanding from our society in terms of their unique cultural and linguistic needs. They are also demanding more linguistically appropriate programmatic interventions, better teachers, and more study abroad programs. They are demanding a stronger emphasis on widening the discussion on the intellectual legacy of thinkers and scholars that historically were not part of the mainstream of the educational system but were part of the cultural backgrounds of the immigrant groups' cultural and linguistic traditions. We can see that in operation in some of the exhibits now more often displayed in museums around the country of the role of indigenous cultures in contemporary societies, the role of the Museum of Barrio in bringing indigenous painters to the public attention, the proliferation of music from different countries, more access through the Internet to linguistically/culturally sensitive literature, the more systematic attempts to develop more culturally and linguistically sensitive instruments of evaluation, etc.

Only a Flexible Model Makes Sense

The more one recognizes the different aspects of bilingual processing and the multiple factors that contribute to the development of the bilingual individual cognitively and emotionally, the more one is forced to consider a flexible model where a variety of factors are operational at different times, depending on the specific needs of the bilingual individuals.

In this model, educational/intervention programs for bilinguals with a subordinate linguistic organization and subordinate linguistic proficiency will be different than for those with a coordinate linguistic organization and balanced proficiency in both languages. Similarly, individuals who already come into the immigration experience with highly developed language and academic skills will require different kinds of interventions. Thus, for instance, "children whose initial level of language proficiency in a single language is highly developed may be in a position to benefit from enrichment bilingual programs while other children have the need for various types of transitional and other bilingual educational programs" (Biakystok & Cummins, 2000, p. 227). It is clear that the social and educational context of the child in the school should be considered when evaluating the effectiveness of the program, the quality of the curriculum, the type of academic skills under consideration, resources, attitude toward the minority language, quality of the instruction, preparation of teachers, and the cognitive and linguistic functioning of the individual.

This model is based on a conceptualization by Bialystok and Cummins (2000) and by Johnson (2000) of the bilingual process, which involves both a central cognitive processing system and linguistic and cognitive operations that can become more specialized in one of the languages. Johnson suggested that some operations may become more specialized in one language because of repeated experience or exposure in that language (like when a bilingual person switches to the first language for mental computation, the language utilized to acquire this operation). They suggest that there is no uniform pattern of development across all operations for bilingual children/individuals or across all bilinguals and that bilingual children may differ from monolingual children in some but not all the constituents of thought, in much the same way that some bilingual children may differ from other bilingual children in the patterns of development (Bialystok & Cummins, 2000).

Thus, we are left with an urgent call for more refined bilingual programs and more systematic research of the kinds suggested by Bialystok (2000), Cummins (1989, 1991, 2000), and Johnson (2000), so as to allow for a more refined understanding of the unique characteristics of bilingual individuals, how they differ in the different domains/skills under consideration, and how they differ from monolingual individuals along multiple cognitive and emotional dimensions.

In the case of evaluation and treatment of the bilingual individuals, similar considerations apply. As indicated earlier, bilingual individuals differ in the way they organize and process their cognitive and affective material and hence evaluators and clinicians should take great care in assessing the specific needs/characteristics of these individuals and design assessment and treatment interventions that take into consideration these qualities. Johnson's model (2000) suggests that each bilingual individual may develop language-specific cognitions, memories, and experiences and that this development is influenced by the kinds of bilingual organization the individual develops and the extent of proficiency acquired in the languages, and the length and nature of experiences in these languages. Thus, for the subordinate bilingual the primary language may be the best language for assessment and treatment, while for the coordinate/compound-proficient bilinguals either language could be utilized, with the understanding that each language may bring about different components of the experience and the material under discussion. What is clear is that any assessment and treatment approach that is universally applied to the bilingual individuals is likely to miss those for whom the approach does not consider their unique bilingual characteristics.

References

Acosta, F. X., & Cristo, M. H. (1981). Development of bilingual interpreter program: An alternative model for Spanish-speaking services. *Professional Psychology, 12*(4), 474–482.

Albert, M., & Obler, L. (1975). *Mixed polyglot aphasia.* Paper at the academy of aphasia. Victoria, B.C. Canada.

Albert, M., & Obler, L. (1978). *The bilingual brain: Neuropsychological and neurolinguistic aspects of bilingualism.* New York: Academic Press.

Ardal, S., Donald, M. W., Meuter, R., Muldrew, S., & Luce, M. (1990). Brain responses to semantic incongruity in bilinguals. *Brain and Language, 39,* 187–205.

Arjona, E. (1977). Intercultural communication and the training of interpreters at the Monterey, institute of foreign studies. In D. Gerver & H. W. Sinaido (Eds.), *Language interpretation and communication.* New York/London: Plenum Press.

Arlow, J. A. (1985). The concept of psychic reality and related problems. *Journal of the American Psychoanalytic Association, 33,* 521–535.

Armour-Thomas, E., & Gopaul-McNicol, S. (1997). In search of correlates of learning underlying "learning disability" using a bio-ecological assessment system. *Journal of Social Distress and the Homeless, 6*(2), 143–159.

Baca, E., & Javier, R. A (1995, July). *El role de los objectos transicionales en el proceso de la separation de la tierra madre: Un estudio realizado con mujeres emigrantes latinas.* Presented at the XXV Interamerican Congress of Psychology, San Juan, Puerto Rico.

Baddeley, A. (1991). *Human memory: Theory and practice.* Hillsdale: Lawrence Erlbaum Associates, Publishers.

Baker, C. (1993). *Foundations of bilingual education and bilingualism.* England: Multilingual Matters Ltd.

Banaji, M. R., & Crowder, R. G. (1989). The bankruptcy of everyday memory. *American Psychologist, 44,* 1185–1193.

Bellak, L., & Faithorn, P. (1981). *Crises and special problems in psychoanalysis and psychotherapy.* New York: Brunner/Mazel.

Bellinger, D., Needleman, H. L., Bromfield, R., & Mintz, M. A. (1986). A follow-up study of the academic attainment and classroom behavior of children with elevated dentine lead levels. *Biol Trace elem Res, 6,* 207–23.

Bernstein, N. (2005, April 21). Language barrier called health hazard in E.R. *The New York Times* (The Metro Section).

Bialystok, E. (Ed.). (2000). Language processing in bilingual children. In E. Bialystok & J. Cummins, *Language, cognition and education of bilingual children* (pp. 222–232). Cambridge: Cambridge University Press.

Bialystok, E. (2001). *Bilingualism in development: Language, literacy, & cognition.* Cambridge: Cambridge University Press.

Bialystok, E. & Cummins, J. (2000). Language, cognition, and education of bilingual children. In E. Bialystok (Ed.), *Language processing in bilingual children* (pp. 222–232). United Kingdom: Cambridge University Press.

Blom, J. P. (1971). Social meaning in linguistic structures: Code-switching in Norway. In J. Gumperz (Ed.), *Language in Social Groups* (pp. 274–310). Stanford, CA: Stanford University Press.

Brenner, C. (1979). The components of psychic conflict and its consequences in mental life. *Psychoanalytic Quarterly, 48,* 547–567.

Brewer, W. F. (1986). What is autobiographical memory? In D. C. Rubin (Ed.), *Autobiographical memory* (pp. 25–49). Cambridge, England: Cambridge University Press.

Bridger, W. H. (1970). The role of cognitive set and stress in generalization of conditional responses to verbal stimuli. *International Journal of Psychobiology, 1,* 39–42.

Brooks, N. (1964). *Language and language learning* (2nd ed.). New York: Harcourt, Bruce & Ward.

Bucci, W. (1985). Dual coding: A cognitive model for psychoanalytic research. *Journal of the American Psychoanalytic Association, 33,* 571–608.

Bucci, W. (1982). The vocalization of painful affect. *Journal of Communication disorders, 15,* 415–440.

Bucci, W. (1997). *Psychoanalysis & cognitive science: A multiple code theory.* New York: Guilford Publications.

Bucci, W., & Freedman, N. (1978). Language and hand: The dimension of referential competence. *Journal of Personality, 46,* 594–622.

Bucci, W., & Freedman, N. (1981). The language of depression. *Bulletin of the Menniger Clinic, 45,* 334–358.

Buxbaum, E. (1949). The role of a second language in the formation of ego and superego. *International Journal of Psychiatry, 18,* 279–289.

Camacho-Ginerich, A. (Ed.). (2002). *Coping in America: The case of the Caribbean East Indians.* New York: The Guyanese East Indian Civic Association.

Cassirer, F. (1953). *Language and myth.* New York: Dover Publications, Inc.

CDC (Centers For Disease Control). (1991). *Preventing lead poisoning in young children: A statement by the Center of Disease Control*, U. S. Department of Health and Human Services, October, 1–64. Atlanta: CDC Report.

Ceci, S. J., & Bronfenbrenner, U. (1991). On the demise of everyday memory: "The rumors of my death are much exaggerated" (Mark Twain). *American Psychologist, 46,* 27–31.

Cenoz, J., & Valencia, J. F. (1994). Additive trilingualism: Evidence from the Basque Country. *Applied Psycho-Linguistics, 15,* 195–207.

Centeno, J. G., & Obler, L. K. (2001). Principles of bilingualism. In M. O. Ponton & J. Leon-Carrión (Eds.), *Neuropsychology and hispanic patient* (pp. 75–86). Mahwah: Lawrence Erlbaum Associates, Publishers.

Chafe, W. L. (Ed.). (1980). *The pear stories-cognitive, cultural, and linguistic aspects of narrative production* (Vol. III). New Jersey: Ablex.

Charlton, M. (1964). Aphasia in bilingual and polyglot patients: A neurological and psychological study. *Journal of Speech and Hearing Disorders, 29,* 307–311.

Chomsky, N. (1957). *Syntactic structures.* The Hague: Mouton & Co.

Chomsky, N. (1965). *Aspects of the theory of syntax.* Cambridge, MA: MIT Press.

Clark, E. (1978). Awareness of language: Some evidence from what children say and do. In A. Sinclair, R. J. Jarvella, & W. J. M. Levelt (Eds.), *The child's concept of language* (pp. 17–44). New York: Springer-Verlang.

Clyne, M. (1967). *Transferring and triggering.* The Hague: Nijhoff.

Cohen G. (1989). *Memory in the real world.* Hillsdale, NJ: Lawrence Erlbaum.

Cohen, G. (1991). *Memory in the real world.* Hillsdale, NJ: Lawrence Erlbaum.

Conway, M. A. (1990a). Associations between autobiographical memories and concepts. *Journal of Experimental Psychology: Learning, Memory and Cognition, 46,* 27–31.

Conway, M. A. (1990b). *Autobiographical memory: An introduction.* Buckingham, England: Open University Press.

Conway, M. A. (1991). In defense of everyday memory. *American Psychologist, 46,* 19–26.

Cooper, R. L (1975). Alternative measures of bilingualism. In J. A. Fishman, R. L. Cooper, & R. Ma (Eds.), *Bilingualism in the Barrio* (pp. 483–512). Bloomington, IN: Indiana University.

Cuellar, I., Arnaldo, B., & Maldonado, R. (1995). Acculturation Rating Scale for Mexican-Americans-II: A revision of the original ARSMA Scale. *Hispanic Journal of Behavioral Sciences, 17*(3), 275–304.

Cummins, J. (1978). Metalinguistic awareness of children in bilingual education programs: Data from Irish and Canadian Ukrainian-English programs. In M. Paradis (Ed.), *Aspects of bilingualism.* Columbia, SC: Hornbeam Press.

Cummins, J. (1986). Empowering minority students: A framework for intervention. *Harvard Educational Review, 56*(1), 18–36.

Cummins, J. (1989). Language and literacy acquisition. *Journal of Multilingual and Multicultural Development, 10*(1), 17–31.

Cummins, J. (1991). The development of bilingual proficiency from home to schools: A longitudinal study of Portuguese speaking children. *Journal of Education, 17*(2), 85–98.

Cummins, J. (2000). Interdependence of first and second language proficiency in bilingual children. In. E. Bialystok (Ed.), *Language processing in bilingual children* (pp. 70–84). Cambridge: Cambridge University Press.

Cummins, J. (Ed.). (2001). Knowledge, power, and identity in teaching English as a second Language. In *Educating second language children: The whole child, the whole curriculum, the whole community.* Cambridge: Cambridge University Press.

Dale, P. S. (1972). *Language development, structure and function.* Hinsdale, IL: Dryden.

Dana, R. H. (1993). *Multicultural assessment perspectives for professional Psychology.* Boston: Allyn & Bacon.

Davis, B. J., & Wertheimer, M. (1967). Some determinants of associations to French and English words. *Journal of Verbal Behavior, 6,* 574–581.

De Groot, A. M. B. (1992a). Bilingual lexical representation: A closer look at conceptual representation. In R. Frost & L. Katz (Eds.), *Orthography, Phonology, Morphology and meaning* (pp. 389–412). Amsterdam: Elsevier Science.

De Groot, A. M. B. (1992b). Determinant of word translations. *Journal of Experimental Psychology: Learning, Memory and Cognition, 18*(5), 1001–1018.

De Groot, A. M. B. (1993). Word-type effects in bilingual processing tasks: Support for a mixed representation system. In R. Schreuder & B. Weltens (Eds.), *The bilingual lexicon* (pp. 27–51). Amsterdam: John Benjamins.

De Zulueta, F. I. S. (1984). The implications of bilingualism in the study and treatment of psychiatric disorders: A review. *Psychological Medicine, 14,* 541–557.

Diebold, A. (1968). The consequences of early bilingualism in cognitive development and personality formation. In E. Norbeck, D. Price-Williams, & W. A. McCord (Eds.),

The study of personality: An interdisciplinary appraisal (pp. 218–245). New York: Holt, Rinehard and Winston.

Diller, K. C. (1974). "Compound" and "coordinate" bilingualism: A conceptual artifact. *Word, 26,* 254–261.

Dubois, B., Levy, R., Verin, M., Teixeira, C., Agid, Y. N., & Pillon, B. (1995). Experimental approach to prefrontal functions in humans. *Annals of the New York Academy of Sciences, 769,* 41–60.

Ellis, A. (2001). *Overcoming destructive beliefs, feelings, and behaviors: New directions for rational emotive behavior therapy.* New York: Prometheus Books.

Ervin, S. (1964). Language and TAT content in bilinguals. *Journal of Abnormal and Social Psychology, 68,* 500–507.

Ervin, S., & Osgood, C. E. (1954). Second language learning and bilingualism. *Journal of Abnormal and Social Psychology, (Supplement), 49,* 139–146.

Fabbro, F., Gran, L. Baso, G., & Brava, A. (1990). Cerebral lateralization in simultaneous interpretation. *Brain and Language, 39,* 69–89.

Fagen, J. W. (1980). Stimulus preference reinforcer effectiveness and relational responding in infants. *Child Development, 51,* 372–378.

Fagen, J. W., Morrongiello, B. S., Rovee-Collien, C. K. S., & Cekoski, M. J. (1984). Expectancies and memory retrieval in three-month old infants. *Child Development, 55,* 936–943.

Fagen, J. W., & Ohr, P. S. (2001). Learning and memory in infancy: Habituation, instrumental conditioning and expectancy formation. In L. T. Singer & P. S. Zeskind (Eds.), *Biobehavioral assessment of the infant* (pp. 233–273). New York: Guilford.

Fagen, J. W., Ohr, P. S., Fleckenstein, L. K. S., & Ribner, D. R. (1985). The effect of crying on long-term memory in infancy. *Child Development, 56,* 1584–1592.

Fagen, J. W., Ohr, P. S., Ribarich, M. I., Klein, S. J., & Adams, P. (1990, April). *Discrimination training, crying and forgetting in young infants.* Paper Presented at TAT Meeting of the Eastern Psychological Association, Philadelphia, PA.

Fagen, J. W., & Prigot, J. A. (1993). Negative affect and infant memory. In C. Rovee-Collier & L. Lipsitt (Eds.), *Advances in infancy research (Vol. 8)* (pp. 169–216). Ablex, NJ: Norwood.

Figueroa, R. A. (1990). Assessment of linguistic minority group children. In C. R. Reynolds & R.W. Kampaus (Eds.), *Handbook of psychological and educational assessment of children (Vol. 1): Intelligence and achievement.* New York: Guilford.

Findling, J. (1969). Bilingual need affiliation and future orientation in extragroup and intragroup domains. *Modern Language-Journal, 53,* 227–231.

Fishman, J. A. (1965). Who speaks what language and to whom and when. *La-Linguistique, 2,* 67–88.

Flanagan, D. P., McGrew, K. S., & Ortiz, S. O. (2000). *The Wechsler intelligence scales and Gf-Gc theory: A contemporary approach to interpretation.* Boston: Allyn & Bacon.

Freedman, N. (1983). On psychoanalytic listening: The construction, paralysis, and reconstruction of meaning. *Psychoanalysis and Contemporary Thought, 6,* 405–434.

Freeman, M. (1985). Psychoanalytic narration and the problem of historical knowledge. *Psychoanalysis and Contemporary Thought, 8,* 133–182.

Friederici, A. (2001). Syntactic, prosodic and semantic processes in the brain: Evidence from event related neuro-imaging. *Journal of Psycholinguistic Research, 30*(3), 237–250.

Freud, S. (1896). The aetiology of hysteria. *Standard Edition, 3,* 189–221.

Freud, S. (1905). Three essays on the theory of sexuality. *Standard Edition, 23,* 255–269.

Freud, S. (1912). Recommendations to physicians practicing psychoanalysis. *Standard Edition, 12,* 109–120.

Freud, S. (1914). On narcissism: An introduction. *Standard Edition, 3,* 189–221.

Freud, S. (1940). An outline of psychoanalysis. *Standard Edition, 23,* 141–207.

Galambos, S. J., & Goldin-Meadow, S. (1990). The effects of learning two languages on levels of metalinguistic awareness. *Cognition, 34,* 1–56.

Gardner, H. (1976). *The shattered mind.* New York: Vintage Books, Random House.

Genesee, F. (Ed.). (2001). *Educating second language children: The whole child, the whole curriculum, the whole community.* Cambridge: Cambridge University Press.

Ginsburg, H., & Opper, S. (1969) *Piaget's theory of intellectual development: An introduction. Englewood cliffs.* New Jersey: Prentice-Hall, Inc.

Goggin, J., & Wickens, D. D. (1971). Proactive interference and language change in short-term memory. *Journal of Verbal Learning and Verbal Behavior, 10,* 453–458.

Goldstein, K. (1948). *Language and language disturbances.* New York: Grune & Stratton.

Gonzalez, I. (2002). *Measuring intelligence in Spanish speaking bilinguals.* Unpublished doctoral dissertation, Ferkauf Graduate School of Psychology, Yeshiva University, New York.

Gonzalez-Reigosa, F. (1976). The anxiety arousing effect of taboo words in bilinguals. In C. D. Spielberger & R. DiazGuerrero (Eds.), *Cross-cultural anxiety.* Washington, DC: Hemisphere Publishing Corp.

Grafman, J. Holyoak, K. J., & Boller, F. (Eds.). (1995). Structure and functions of the human prefrontal cortex. *Annals of the New York Academy of Sciences, 769,* 1–410.

Greenfield, L., & Fishman, J. A. (1975). Situational measures of normative language views of persons, place and topic among Puerto Rican bilinguals. In J. A. Fishman, R. L. Cooper, & R. Ma (Eds.), *Bilingualism in the Barrio* (pp. 233–252). Bloomington, IN: Indiana University.

Greenson, R. (1950). The mother tongue and the mother. *International Journal of Psychiatry, 31,* 18–23.

Grosjean, F. (1982) *Life with two languages: An introduction to bilingualism.* Cambridge, MA: Harvard University Press.

Grosjean, F. (1989). Neurolinguists, beware! The bilingual is not two monolinguals in one person. *Brain and Language, 36,* 3–15.

Hahne, A. (2001). What's different in second-language processing? Evidence from event-related brain potentials. In Special issue: Brain imaging and sentence processing. *Journal of Psycholinguistic Research, 30*(3), 251–266.

Hahne, A., & Friedirici, A. D. (2001). Processing a second language: Late learners comprehension mechanisms as revealed by event-related brain potentials. *Bilingualism: Language and Cognition, 4*(2), 123–141.

Halpern, L. (1941). Beitrag zur Restitution der aphasie bei polylotton in Hinblich auf das Hebraeische. *Schweizer Archiv fuer Neurologie and Psychiatrie, 47,* 150–154.

Helms, J. (2003, February). *How to use black racial identity theory to solve the black-white test score gap.* Presented at the 20th anniversary of Winter Roundtable Identity in cultural Psychology and Education, Columbia University.

Hines, T. (1978, August). *Bilingual memory: Independent, interdependent, or both? Paper presented at the Annual Meeting of the American Psychological Association,* Toronto, Canada.

Hoover, M. L. (1992). Sentence processing strategies in Spanish and English. *Journal of Psycholinguistic Research, 21*(4), 275–299.

Hornby, P. A. (1977). *Bilingualism: An introduction and overview.* In P. A. Hornby (Ed.), *Bilingualism: Psychological, social ad educational implications.* New York: Academic Press.

Hull, R. A. (2003). *How does bilingualism matter? A meta-analytic tale of two hemispheres.* Unpublished doctoral dissertation, A&M University, Texas.

Imoff, G. (1990). The position of the US English on bilingual education. In C. B. Cazden and C. E. Snow (Eds.), *The annals of the American academy of political & social science 508* (pp. 48–61), London: Sage.

Isham, W. P., & Lane, H. (Winter, 1994). A common conceptual code in bilingualism: Evidence from simultaneous interpretation. *Sign Language Studies 85*, 291–316.

Jacobovits, L., & Lambert, W. (1961). Semantic satiation among bilinguals. *Journal of Experimental Psychology, 62,* 576–582.

Javier, R. A. (1989), Linguistic consideration in the treatment of bilinguals. *Psychoanalytic Psychology, 6,* 87–96.

Javier, R. A. (1995). Vicissitudes of autobiographical memories in bilingual analysis. *Psychoanalytic Psychology, 12,* 429–438.

Javier, R. A. (1996). Psychodynamic treatment with the urban poor. In R. P. Foster, M. Moskowitz, & R. A. Javier (Eds.), *Reaching across boundaries of culture and class: Widening the scope of psychotherapy* (pp. 93–113). Northvale, NJ, London: Jason Aronson, Inc.

Javier, R. A., & Alpert, M. (1986). The effect of stress on the linguistic generalization of coordinate bilinguals. *Journal of Psycholinguistic Research, 15,* 419–435.

Javier, R. A., Barroso, F., & Muñóz, M. (1993), Autobiographical memory in bilinguals. *Journal of Psycholinguistic Research, 2,* 319–338.

Javier, R. A., & Camacho-Gingerich, A. (2004). Risk and resilience in the Latino youth. In C. S. Clauss-Ehlers & M. D. Weist (Eds.), *Community planning to foster resilience in children* (pp. 65–82). New York: Kluwer Academic/Plenum Publishers.

Javier, R. A., & Marcos, L. R. (1989). The role of stress on the language-independence and code-switching phenomena. *Journal of Psycholinguistic Research, 18,* 449, 472.

Javier, R. A., Vasquez, C. I., & Marcos, L. R. (1998). Common errors by interpreters in communicating with linguistically diverse patients. In R. A. Javier & W. H. Herron (Eds.), *Personality development and psychotherapy in our diverse society: A sourcebook* (pp. 521–534). Northdale, NJ: Jason Aronson, Inc.

Johnson, J. (2000). Contructive processes in bilingualism and their cognitive growth effects. In E. Bialystok (Ed.), *Language processing in bilingual children* (pp. 193–221). Cambridge: Cambridge University Press.

Jones, B. P. (1993), Repression: The evolution of a psychoanalytic concept from the 1890's to the 1990's. *Journal of the American Psychoanalytic Association, 41,* 63–93.

Karmiloff-Smith, A. (1986). Stage/structure versus phase/process in modeling linguistic and cognitive development. In I. Levin (Ed.), *Stage and structure: Re-opening the debate.* Norwood, NJ: Ablex Press.

Karpov, Y. V., & Haywood, H. C. (1998). Two ways to elaborate Vygotsky's concept of mediation - Implications for instruction. *American Psychologist, 53*(1), 27–36.

Kimmel, H. D., Pendergrass, V. E., & Kimmel, E. B. (1967). Modifying children's orienting reactions instrumentally. *Conditioning Reflex, 2,* 2–27.

Kirsner, K., Smith, M. C., Lockhart, R. S., King, M. L., & Jain, M. (1984). The bilingual lexicon: Language-specific units in an integrated network. *Journal of Verbal Learning and Verbal Behavior, 23,* 519–539.

Kohut, H. (1977). *The restoration of the self.* New York: International University Press.

Kolers, P. A. (1963). Interlingual word associations. *Journal of Verbal Learning and Verbal Behavior, 2,* 291–300.

Kolers, P. A. (1968). Bilingualism and information processing. *Scientific American, March,* 79–86.

Kolers, P. A., & Paradis, M. (1980). Psychological and linguistic studies of bilingualism. *Canadian Journal of Psychology, 34,* 287–305.

Krapf, E. E. (1955). The choice of language in polyglot psychoanalysis. *Psychoanalytic Quarterly, 24,* 343–357.

Lambert, W. (1972). *Language, psychology and culture* (pp. 330–331). Stanford, CA: Stanford University Press.

Lambert, W. (1955). Measurement of linguistic dominance of bilinguals. *Journal of Abnormal and Social Psychology, 50,* 197–200.

Lambert W., & Fillenbaum, S. (1959). A pilot study of aphasia among bilinguals. *Canadian Journal of Psychology, 13,* 28–34.

Lambert W., Havelka, J., & Crosby, C. (1958) The influence of language-acquisition contexts on bilingualism. *Journal of Abnormal and Social Psychology, 19k.* 56, 239–244.

Lambert, W. E., Ignatow, M., & Krauthamier, M. (1968). Bilingual organization in free-recall. *Journal of Verbal Learning and Verbal Behavior, 7,* 207–214.

Lehrer, W., & Sloan, J. (2005). *Crossing the BLVD: Strangers, neighbors, aliens in a new America.* New York/London: Norton & Company.

Leischner, A. (1948). Ueber die aphasie der Mehrsprachigen. *Archiv fuer Psychiatrie and Nervenkrankheiten, 180,* 118–180, 731–775.

Lenneberg, E. (1967). *Biological foundation of language.* New York: Wiley.

L'Hermitte, R., Hecaen, H., Dubois, J., Culioli, A., & Tabouret-Keller, A. (1966). Le probleme de l'aphasie des polygottes: Remargues sur quelques observations. *Neurolopsychologia, 4,* 315–329.

Lipski, J. M. (1978). Code-Switching and the problem of language competence. In M. Paradis (Ed.), *Aspect of bilingualism* (pp 250–264). Durham, SC: Hornbeam Press, Inc.

Locke, J. L. (1994). Phases in the child's development of language. *American Scientist, 82,* 436–445.

Loftus, E. F. (1979). *Eyewitness testimony.* Cambridge, MA: Harvard University Press.

Longley, P. (1977). An integrated programme for training interpreters. In D. Gerver & H. W. Sinaido (Eds.), *Language interpretation and communication.* New York/London: Plenum Press.

Lopez, S., & Nuñez, J. A. (1987). Cultural factors considering in selected diagnostic criteria and interview schedules. *Journal of Abnormal Psychology, 96,* 270–272.

Lopez, M., & Young, R. M. (1974). The linguistic interdependence of bilinguals. *Journal of Experimental Psychology, 102,* 981–983.

Luria, A. (1973). *The working brain: An introduction to neuropsychology.* New York: Basic Books, Inc. Publisher.

Luria, A. (1981). *Language and cognition.* Washington, DC: Winston.

Luria, A., & Vinogradova, O. (1959). Objective investigation of the dynamicsof semantic systems. *British Journal of Psychology, 50,* 89.

Luria, A., & Yudovich, F. (1968). *Speech and the development of the mental processes in the child.* London: Staples Press.

Lyman, R., Kwan, S., & Chao, W. (1938). Left occiptio-parietal brain tumor. *The Chinese Medical Journal, 54,* 491–516.

Mackey, W. F. (1962). The description of bilingualism. *Canadian Journal of Linguistics, 6,* 51–85.

Macnamara, J. (1967). How can one measure the extent of a person's bilingual proficiency? In L. Kelly (Ed.), *Description and measurement of bilingualism: An international seminar, University of Moncton,* June 6–14 (pp. 80–99). Toronto. Toronto: University of Toronto Press.

Macnamara, J., & Kushnir, S. L. (1971). Linguistic independence of bilinguals. The input switch. *Journal of Verbal Learning and Verbal Behavior, 10,* 480–487.

Mahler, M. S., Pine, F., & Bergman, A. (1975). *The psychological birth of the human infant.* New York: Basic Books.

Marcos, L. M. (1989). Effects of interpreters on the evaluation of psychopathology in non-English-speaking patients. *American Journal of Psychiatry, 136*(2), 171–174.

Marcos, L. R. (1976). Bilinguals in psychotherapy: Languge as an emotional barrier. *American Journal of Psychotherapy, 30,* 552–560.

Marcos, L. R., & Alpert, M. (1976). Strategies and risks in psychotherapy with bilingual patients: The phenomenon of language independence. *American Journal of Psychiatry, 133,* 1275–1278.

Marcos, L. R., Alpert, M., Urcuyo, L., & Kesselman, M. (1973). The effect of interview language on the evaluation of psychopathology in Spanish-American schizophrenic patients. *American Journal of Psychiatry, 130,* 540–553.

Marin, G., Sabogal, F. Marin, B., Otero-Sabogal, R., & Perez-Stable, E. J. (1987). Development of a short acculturation scale for Hispanics. *Hispanic Journal of Behavioral Sciences, 9,* 183–205.

Mcormack, P. D. (1977). *Bilingual linguistic memory: The independence-interdependence issues and educational implications.* New York: Academic Press.

Miller, J. (1991, September 15). Strangers at the gate. *The New York Times Magazine,* 32–37, 49, 80–81.

Nair, K. R., & Virmani, V. (1973). Speech and language disturbances on hemisplegia. *Indian Journal-of-Medical Research, 61,* 1395–1403.

Namy, C. (1977). Relections on the training of simultaneous interpreters: A metalinguistic approach. In D. Gerver & H. W. Sinaido (Eds.), *Language interpretation and communication.* London: Plenum Press.

Needleman, H. L., Schell, A., Bellinger, D., Leviton, A., & Allred, E. N. (1990). The long-term effects of exposure to low doses of lead in childhood: An 11-year follow-up report. *The NEW England Journal of Medicine, 322,* 83–88.

Neisser, U., Boodow, G., Bouchard, T. J., Boykin, A. W., Brody, N., Ceci, S. J., Halpern, D. F., Loghlin, J. C., Perloff, R., Sternberg, R. J., & Surbina, S. (1996). Intelligence: Knowns and unknowns. *American Psychologists, 51,* 77–101.

NPR-National Public Radio, 3/16/02.

Obler, L. K. & Albert, M. (1977). Influence of aging on recovery from aphasia in polyglots. *Brain and Language, 4,* 460–463.

Obler, L. K., Centeno, J., & Eng, N. (1995). Bilingual and polyglot aphasia. In L. Menn, M. O'Connor, L. K. Obler, & A. Holland (Eds.), *Non-fluent aphasia in a multilingual world.* (pp. 132–143). Amsterdam: John Benjamin Publishing Company.

Ojemann, G. A., & Whitaker, H. A. (1978). The bilingual brain. *Archives of Neurology,* 35, 409–412.

Osgood, C. E. (1952). The nature and measurement of meaning. *Psychological Bulletin, 49,* 197–237.

Paradis, M. (1978).The stratification of bilingualism. In M. Paradis (Ed.), *Aspects of bilingualism* (pp. 165–175). Durham SC: Hornbeam Press, Inc.
Paradis, M. (1983). *Readings on aphasia in bilinguals and polyglots.* Montreal: Didier.
Paradis, M. (1993). Multilingualism and aphasia. In G. Blankin et al. (Eds.), *Linguistics disorders and pathologies* (pp. 278–288). Berlin: De Gruyter.
Paradis, M. (1994). Neurolinguistic aspects of implicit and explicit memory: Implications for bilinguilism. In N. Ellis (Ed.), *Implicit and explicit learning of second language* (pp. 343–419). London: Academic Press.
Paradis, M. (2003). The bilingual Loch Ness Monster raises its non-asymmetric head again-or, why bother with such cumbersome notions as validity and reliability? Comments on Evans et al. (2002). *Brain and Language, 87,* 441–448.
Paradis, M. (2004, May). Personal E-Mail Communication.
Paz, O. (1970). Traduccion: Literatura y Literalidad. *Cuadernos Marginales, 18,* 7–19.
Penfield, W., & Roberts, L. (1959). *Speech and brain mechanisms.* Princeton, NJ: Princeton University Press.
Perani, D., Paulesu, F., Galles, N. S., Dupoux, E., Dehaene, S., Bettinardi, V. et al. (1998). The bilingual brain proficiency and age of acquisition of 10 second languages, *Brom, 121,* 1841–1852.
Peraino, K., & Thomas, E. (2002). Odyssey into Jihad. Newsweek, January 14, pp. 40–48.
Perez-Foster, R. M. (1992). Psychoanalysis and bilingual patient: Some observations on the influence of language choice on transference. *Psychoanalytic Psychology, 9,* 61–76
Perez-Foster, R. M. (1996). Assessing the psychodynamic function of language in bilingual patient. In R. M. Perez-Foster, M. Moskowitz, & R. A. Javier (Eds.), *Reading across boundaries of culture and class* (pp. 246–263), Northvale, NJ: Jason Aronson, Inc.
Petrides, M. (1995). Functional organization of the human prefrontal cortex for mneumonic processing: Evidence from neuroimaging studies. *Annals of the New York Academic of Sciences, 769,* 85–96.
Piaget, J. (1954). *The construction of reality in the child.* New York: Basic Books.
Piaget, J. (1980). *Experiments in contradiction.* Chicago: University of Chicago
Piaget, J. (1995). *The language and thought of the child.* Cleveland: Meridan.
Pitres, A. (1895). Etude su l' aphasie. *Revue de Medecine, 15,* 873–899.
Pope, B., Blass, T., Siegman, A. W., & Raher, J. (1970). Anxiety and depression in speech. *Consulting and Clinical Psychology, 35,* 128–133.
Quiñones, M. E. (2007). Bridging the Gap. In J. C. Muran (Ed.), *Dialogues on differece: Studies of diversity in the therapeutic relationship* (pp. 153–167). Washington, DC: American Psychological Association.
Rapport, R. L., Tan, C. T., & Whitaker, H. A. (1983). Language function and dysfunction among Chinese-and English- speaking polyglots: Cortical stimulation, Wada testing, and clinical studies. *Brain and Language, 18,* 342–366.
Razran, G. H. S. (1939). A quantitative study of meaning by a conditioned salivary technique (semantic conditioning). *Science, 90,* 89–90.
Redlinger, W. (1976). A description of transference and code-switching. In G. D. Keller, R.V. Teschner, & S. Viera (Eds.), *Bilingualism in the bicentennial and beyond* (pp. 41–52). New York: Editorial Bilingue.
Reik, T. (1958). *Listening with the third Ear: The inner experience of a psychoanalyst.* New York: Farrar, Straus.
Ribot, T. (1882). *Diseases of memory: An essay in the positive psychology.* London: Paul.
Riccio, D. C., Rabinowitz, V. C., & Axerold, S. (1994). Memory: when less is more. *American Psychologist, 49*(11), 917–926.

Rieber, R. W., & Wollock, J. (Eds.) (1997). *The collected works of L. S. Vygotsky: Volume 3, Problems of the theory and history of psychology* (R. Van Der Veer, Trans.). New York: Plenum Press.

Riess, B. (1940). Semantic conditioning involving the Galvanic Skin Reflex. *Journal of Experimental Psychology, 26,* 238–240.

Rubin, J. (1962). Bilingualism in Paraguay. *Anthropological Linguistics, 4*(1), 52–58.

Schachtel, E. G. (1947). On memory and childhood amnesia. *Psychiatry, 10,* 1–26.

Schacter, E. G., Kagan, J., & Leichtman, M. D (1995). True and false memories in children and adults: A cognitive neuroscience perspective. *Psychology, Public Policy, and Law, 1*(2), 411–428.

Schlachet, E. G., & Aragno, A. (1994, March). *The accessibility of early experience through the language of origin: A theoretical integration.* Paper presented at the Seventh Biennial Conference, the Psychoanalytic Society of the Postdoctoral Program, New York University.

Schneider, H. L. (1981). *The language independence phenomenon and emotional expression in coordinate bilinguals.* Unpublished doctoral dissertation, New York University.

Schnitzer, M. L. (1978). Cerebral lateralization and plasticity: Their relevance to language acquisition. In M. Paradis (Ed.), *Aspects of bilingualism* (pp. 1–49). Durham, SC: Hornbeam Press, Inc.

Schrauf, R. W. (2000). Bilingual autobiographical memory: Experimental studies and clinical cases. *Culture & Psychology, 6,* 387–417.

Shaffer, D. (1978). The place of code-switching in linguistic contacts. In M. Paradis (Ed.), *Aspects of bilingualism* (pp. 265–274). Durham, SC: Hornbeam Press, Inc.

Smith, M. C. (1991). On the recruitment of semantic information of the word fragment: Evidence from the bilingual priming. *Journal of Experimental Psychology: Learning, Memory, and Cognition, 17*(2), 234–244.

Snow, C. (1981). *English speakers' acquisition of Dutch syntax: Comparisons of first and second language.* Paper presented at the Conference on native language and foreign language acquisition, New York.

Sollee, N. A. (1963). *A study of perceptual defense involving bilinguals: An experiment.* Unpublished Master's thesis, University of Philippines.

Stengel, E. (1939). On learning a new language. *International Journal of Psychiatry, 20,* 471–479.

Sullivan, H. S. (1953). *The interpersonal theory of psychiatry.* New York: Norton.

Tallal, P., Galaburda, A. M., Llinás, R. R., & Euler, C. V. (Eds.) (1993). Temporal information processing in the nervous system. *Annals of the New York Academy of Sciences, 682,* 1–439.

Thorson, G. (1980, September). *Interlingual priming effects in bilinguals.* Paper presented at the annual meeting of the American Psychological Association, Montreal, Canada.

Time-Special report (2001 November 12). Inside Al-Qaeda: Bin Laden's web of terror Time, December 3, 2001.

Monterey, C. A. (1975). GSR biofeedback in psychotherapy: Some clinical observations. *Psychotherapy: Theory, Research and Practice, 12,* 33–38.

Tulving, E., & Calotta, V. A. (1970). Free recall of trilingual lists. *Cognitive Psychology, 1,* 86–98.

US Census Bureau, 2000/2002

Vaid, J., & Menon, R. (2000). Correlates of Bilinguals' preferred Language for mental computations. *SAL, 4*(2), 325–342.

Valdes, F. G. (1976). Social interaction and code-switching patterns: A case study of Spanish/English alternatives. In G. D Keller, R. V Teschner, & S. Viera (Eds.), *Bilingualism in the bicentennial and beyond* (pp. 53–85). New York: Editorial Bilingue.

Vasquez, C. A., & Javier, R. A. (1991). The problem with interpreters: Communicating with Spanish-speaking patients. *Hospital and Community Psychiatry, 42*(2), 163–165.

Vygotsky, L. S. (1962). *Thought and language.* Cambridge, MA: MIT Press. (Originally published in 1934.)

Wagenaar, W. (1986). My memory: A study of autobiographical memory over six years. *Cognitive Psychology, 18,* 225–252.

Wakefield, J. A., Bradley, P. E., Byong-Hee, Yom, & Doughtie, E. B. (1975). Language-switching and constituent structure. *Language and Speech, 18,* 14–19.

Wallerstein, R. S. (1985). The concept of psychic reality: Its meaning and value. *Journal of the American Psychoanalytic Association, 33,* 555–569.

Weber-Fox, C. M., & Neville, H. J. (1996). Maturational constraints on functional specializations for language processing: ERP and behavioral evidence in bilingual speakers. *Journal of Cognitive Neuroscience, 8,* 231–256.

Wechsler, A. (1977). Dissociative alexia. *Archives of Neurology, 34,* 2–57.

Weingartner, H. (1978). Human state-dependent learning. In B. T. Ho, D. W. Richards, & D. C. Chute (Eds.), *Drug discrimination and state-dependent learning* (pp. 361–382). New York: Academic Press.

Weinreich, U. (1953). *Languages in contact: Findings and problems.* The Hague: Mouton.

Welles, J. K. (1993, April). *Counterfeit analyses. Maintaining the illusion of knowing.* Paper presented at the meeting of the American Psychological Association Division 39, New York.

Whorf, B. (1956). *Language, thoughts and reality.* Cambridge: M.I.T. Press.

Winnicott, D. W. (1965). *The maturational processes and the facilitating environment.* New York: International Universities Press.

Winograd, E., & Killinger, W. A. (1983). Relating age at encoding in early childhood to adult recall: Development of flashbulb memories. *Journal of Experimental Psychology: General, 112,* 413–422.

Wolff, P. H. (1988). The real and reconstructed past. *Psychoanalysis and Contemporary Thought, 11,* 379–414.

Index

Printed in the United States
82351LV00002BA/142

9 780387 309132